# THE HEALING ART
## OF
# TAI CHI

*Becoming One with Nature*

# THE HEALING ART
## OF
# TAI CHI

## *Becoming One with Nature*

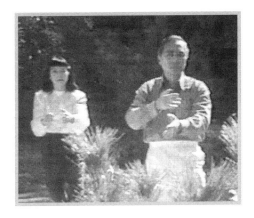

Martin J. Lee, PhD

Emily Lee, TC Master

Joyce Lee & Melinda Lee

**World Scientific**

NEW JERSEY · LONDON · SINGAPORE · BEIJING · SHANGHAI · HONG KONG · TAIPEI · CHENNAI · TOKYO

*Published by*

World Scientific Publishing Co. Pte. Ltd.

5 Toh Tuck Link, Singapore 596224

*USA office:* 27 Warren Street, Suite 401-402, Hackensack, NJ 07601

*UK office:* 57 Shelton Street, Covent Garden, London WC2H 9HE

**British Library Cataloguing-in-Publication Data**
A catalogue record for this book is available from the British Library.

**THE HEALING ART OF TAI CHI**
**Becoming One with Nature**

ISBN 978-981-3271-88-3
ISBN 978-981-3273-08-5 (pbk)

For any available supplementary material, please visit
https://www.worldscientific.com/worldscibooks/10.1142/11032#t=suppl

Typeset by Stallion Press
Email: enquiries@stallionpress.com

Printed in Singapore

# Dedication

To Bo for being a model for us with his great vision, willpower, physical strength, and entrepreneurial spirit; to James for his love and devotion to his family and the scholarly and intellectual influence he imparted to us; to Susanne for her great virtues and kindness; and to Mu Kin for her faith in education and spiritual support.

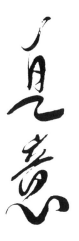

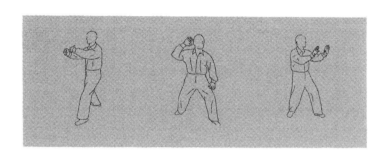

# Contents

# Acknowledgments

We are grateful for the help of many friends, students, and family members who participated in the various preparation stages of this book. Our special thanks go to Robert Shepard, who encouraged us to write a sequel to our first book on tai chi, co-authored with JoAn Johnstone, *Ride the Tiger to the Mountain; T'ai Chi for Health* (1989). He has provided valuable comments and suggestions helpful in creating this new book.

We would like to thank our friend Lynn Hunton for his ingenious creation of the multi-image photos of the tai chi movements and for his painstaking efforts and patience in shooting and developing these unique photos. Also, thank you to Martha Hunton for helping us with the cover for the first edition of this book and for her creative insights.

Our special love goes to Criss for her help with the manuscript and to Bryce and Bessie for their interest, ideas, feedback, and support in organizing and writing this book.

We are also indebted to Dr. Robert Kahn for writing the preface and for taking part in self-healing experiments. We thank John Hughes and Jerry Harp for sharing their tai chi stories and Dr. Steve St. Lorant and Mrs. Lilo St. Lorant for providing enlightening quotes.

# A Tai Chi Fable

*A tai chi master came to the village to catch a tiger. Upon finding the tiger, the master looked into the tiger's eyes. Without any struggle, the tiger fell to his knees. The master sat on the tiger's back and rode the tiger to the mountain. While sitting on the back of the tiger, the master attained enlightenment. Thereafter, the master returned from the mountain to help others become one with nature.*

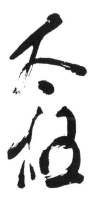

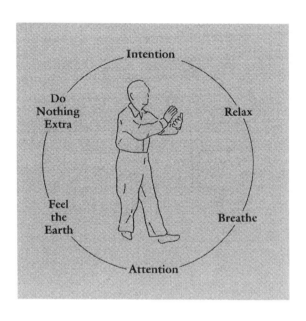

# Preface

My decision to learn tai chi was casual, almost accidental. My decision to continue learning and to practice it regularly, however, is firm and deliberate. This book demonstrates the reasons for that decision.

About a year ago, my wife and I joined a beginners' class in tai chi taught by Martin and Emily Lee. Friends of ours had already enrolled, hoping to get relief from arthritic symptoms and improvement in balance. We went along with them, partly to offer companionship and partly out of curiosity. My expectations were for some calesthenic exercises, no more.

The tai chi movements were interesting in themselves, easy and graceful when our instructors did them, awkward and uncertain when we attempted to follow them. Practice brought improvement. Nevertheless, when Martin Lee occasionally asked members of the class whether, at some appropriate point in the exercise sequence, they had felt *ch'i*, the flow of energy or inner breath that tai chi is designed to evoke, my answer was always no.

Moreover, I was extremely skeptical about the concept itself, which is so different from what little physiology I knew. But I was intrigued by Martin's four basic instructions as we practiced the tai chi moves: Relax, breathe, feel the earth, and do nothing extra.

My fascination with these four principles was both pragmatic and intellectual. The pragmatic aspect was sheer surprise at the difficulty of keeping the four points in mind as I practiced the moves. It was a discovery to learn that I unconsciously tensed up in preparation for a move, held my breath, locked my knees, and hunched my shoulders. All four principles violated almost automatically!

The intellectual interest came as I began to think of other ancient cultures that had, in their own ways, come to similar insights and had embodied them in myth and religion. I remembered the Greek story of Antaeus, the giant son of mother earth (Gaia), who was invincible only as long as his feet remained in touch with the ground. I thought of the Delphic oracle, whose supreme admonition to each human being was "Know thyself." When Martin spoke of tai chi as a way of becoming one with nature, I thought of the Navajo way, the concept of health as harmony of the person with nature, and of illness as no longer walking in harmony.

My skepticism received its first shock one afternoon when, in the process of doing the Grand Tai Chi, I felt the sense of warmth that Martin had described as the flow of ch'i. I cannot reproduce it at will and yet I cannot doubt the sensation. I did not know whether to attribute it to ch'i, however, or to some kind of self-hypnotic effect of my own suggestibility.

Before I had resolved this issue to my satisfaction, I had a much more dramatic example of the effect of ch'i—its power to heal or, more properly, to enable the individual to heal. When Martin had told me about this, I had responded with doubt and with some mention of the placebo effect. He invited me to observe the process one evening, when he offered to teach self-healing to any member of his tai chi class who had troubling physical symptoms.

I came with a brief questionnaire in which people described their pain, explained its apparent cause, and rated its severity. I observed and timed the procedure which Martin demonstrated and each person imitated. I asked each one to rate the intensity of the pain after this self-treatment, on the same scale they had used before it.

The results were astounding—to them and to

me. A woman whose head movement had been severely limited since an automobile accident showed almost normal range of movement within 30 minutes. Another person, who had a marked swelling in one hand after a fall, was able to reduce the swelling almost to normal. And so it went, person after person, all evening. I observed, timed, questioned, and continued to doubt—not what I had seen but the reasons for it.

Martin Lee, amiable as always, only said that it was unfortunate that I had no symptom of my own, so that I could experience directly as well as observe. At that point, my wife said what I had refused to admit—that I had mentioned a persistent shoulder pain since changing a tire about two weeks earlier, not severe, but enough to make me avoid lifting with that arm or sleeping on that side of my body.

I thus became subject as well as observer, and I can only report that the pain, which had persisted unchanged for more than two weeks, vanished within 20 minutes. Moreover, it has not re- turned. Martin and I have discussed these effects in terms that are more easily accepted by Western science. Many pains are compound: a combination of an initial trauma and the compensatory distortions and spasms which we adopt, often unconsciously, to protect the damaged area. When the relaxing procedure does its work, these painful secondary effects are relieved.

I find this explanation helpful but not adequate to account for what I have observed and experienced. This book is an attempt by Martin Lee, offered with characteristic candor, to provide a more complete explanation. It invites openness of mind, openness to new ways of thinking. It is exploratory rather than doctrinaire, and it invites the reader to join the exploration and thus to obey the Delphic admonition: "Know thyself."

Dr. Robert L. Kahn
Professor Emeritus of Psychology
and Public Health
University of Michigan, Ann Arbor

# East Meets West
## *How I Came to Tai Chi*

❧

Both Eastern and Western cultures have influenced my life, sculpting and defining who I am. Born and reared in China, I came to the United States at 16, enticed by its opportunities. Since my parents taught me that education was an important factor for determining my future, I worked to excel in the sciences and philosophy.

I came from a family of traditional Chinese scholars. I remember sitting, at age 4, on my great-grandfather's lap and playing with his long whiskers while he read poetry and recited sayings from Confucius. My great-grandfather, who had passed the first civil service exams at the end of the Ching dynasty, had become a "national scholar" after passing one of three. But the Nationalist government discarded such civil service exams; so, he had been unable to pursue a career as a civil servant as his ancestors had.

Since I was brought up in China in a time of war and chaos, confusion and reform, getting a solid education was not easy. As war enveloped the country, my family moved to an unoccupied area of China so that I could continue my schooling. After the war, when I was in high school, I moved to Hong Kong and lived in my great-grandfather's room. I dreamed of becoming a poet and philosopher like him.

On my 16th birthday, I arrived in San Francisco, and not long afterward, my grandfather took me to visit the University of California campus at Berkeley. When I saw an automatic door opener at the school of engineering, I was so impressed that I decided to study science and engineering. Two years later, I entered Berkeley's electrical engineering school, majoring in engineering and physics. I also studied Chinese philosophy and poetry. Dr. Peter Broodberg, who taught Taoist and Confucian philosophy, and Dr. Thomas Everhart, who taught microwave fields, inspired and encouraged me and had a tremendous impact on my life.

As a student, I suffered from severe hay fever and asthma attacks which caused me much pain. Eventually I was hospitalized. After tests, I discovered that I was allergic to molds, dust, and pollens.

After graduation, I moved to New Jersey to work at the Bell Telephone Laboratories and to attend New York University, where I earned a master's in electrical engineering. At Bell I acquired hands-on experience in microwave measurements. Then I moved back to California to work at the Stanford Linear Accelerator Center (SLAC) at Stanford University.

I had thought that leaving New Jersey and moving back to California would relieve my allergies, but they got worse and I underwent a regimen of allergy shots and other treatments. As I began work on my doctorate at Stanford while working full-time and rearing a young family, my condition steadily worsened. I often wore a mask over my mouth and lay on a couch with an electronic air cleaner blowing at me. Since modern medicine had failed me I turned to tai chi.

Under Tai Chi Master Kuo Lien-Yin, I began practicing tai chi and my condition gradually improved. Eventually, I recovered completely even though my work life remained stressful. I was working on the design of a particle storage ring, called the Stanford Positron Electron Assymetric

Ring (SPEAR), under my doctoral thesis adviser, Dr. Burton Richter. SPEAR was operated by a computer model, using a method I developed. Today, all modern accelerators use this same computer-model-based method. So, I became a sort of guru of particle accelerators.

Using SPEAR a team of scientists led by Dr. Richter discovered the psi atomic particle at the Stanford Linear Accelerator Center, which revealed the secret hidden inside the atomic nuclei. In 1976 Dr. Richter and Dr. Samuel Chao Chung Ting, at Massachusetts Institute of Technology, shared a Nobel Prize in physics for this discovery.

Physics and math teaches me to be logical and systematic. As an engineer and scientist, I attempt to analyze and solve problems rationally. I also accept only things that I can see and understand and question those that I cannot see and understand. The early excitement in my career had not allowed me to forget the asthma and allergies that had nearly derailed my studies. I wondered about the healing process of tai chi, which had seemed miraculous, and began teaching tai chi at a community center with my wife, Emily, who is also a tai chi master.

As I taught Tai Chi for Total Fitness, I began to see the healing power of tai chi at work on my students. So, I decided to study the relationship between wellness and the four parts of the self—mind, body, thought, and ch'i (inner energy).

The Chinese, who have written about ch'i for centuries, have suggested that ch'i kung (qi-gong), a system of breathing exercises to enhance healing, was invented by an emperor 3,500 years ago. Chinese acupuncture, martial arts like tai chi, and meditation have emerged in part from the study of ch'i and ch'i-related exercises.

But I did not fully understand the role of ch'i in the healing process until I studied ch'i kung with Dr. Yu Pen-Shih. Dr. Yu, a distinguished physician and ch'i kung master famous in China, came at my invitation to Stanford and lived with us two years. Dr. Yu had also been a chosen disciple of a living Buddha, Chie Shung Master. (*Chie* means "uphold" and *Shung* means "pine

tree," a symbol of longevity.) Emily and I were fortunate enough to become his only Buddhist students in America.

By practicing tai chi and understanding ch'i and its breathing techniques, I was able to heal my allergies and other ailments. I hadn't lost my interest in philosophy from my early college days. So, I began to combine Western science and Eastern philosophy in what I call *physical philosophy,* connecting what I felt to be important contributions to knowledge from both East and West. Through this physical philosophy I have gained greater appreciation of science, philosophy, God, and nature. I hope you achieve greater happiness and good health through the physical philosophy I present in this book.

Today we have acquired considerable scientific knowledge about the universe and the world immediately around us. We can travel in space, direct atoms to create energy, alter DNA, and develop an information superhighway. Although all these inventions may give us the advantage of living better and longer, for many of us pain and suffering are still a part of everyday life. Why? Because of stress.

The stress we feel as individuals creates an enormous emotional and spiritual burden on society. People afflicted with stress rarely seek a cure, supposing that stress is not detrimental to health. But there is growing evidence that stress contributes to devastating physical and mental ailments. When we're under stress, we lose control of our lives, and this loss of control makes us even more "stressed out." Unless we find ways to reduce this stress, most of us experience anger, worry, and sorrow, sometimes for an extended time. This residual stress in turn can cause headaches, other physical complaints, and depression. If we want to enjoy a better life, we need to find ways to reduce and, better yet, to prevent stress. Preventing stress from accumulating keeps it from harming the body and mind and debilitating our energy.

Many experts have discussed the links between mind and body and the need to prevent stress, but few have offered a systematic, effective, and manageable way to restore both body and mind to their natural, stress-free state. Although I once suffered from the physical manifestations of stress, I was able to cure these ailments through the practice of tai chi. As a tai chi master and "physical philosopher," I combined Western science and Eastern philosophy in my study of the causes of stress. The best solution I've found is tai chi.

In my 20 years of teaching tai chi, I looked at students' physical ailments that could be traced to stress and considered possible causes. It seemed simple. We're living in a society that has become out of touch with nature. Consider the words of the 6th century Chinese philosopher Lao Tze.

"The intelligent person is like a little child. The child's vitality is intact, the child's existence is harmonious. To enjoy such harmony is to be in accord with nature. To be in accordance with nature is to be achieving the goal of life."

After realizing how much my students' cases had in common, I developed a simple yet effective method, based on the principles of tai chi, to overcome both symptoms and causes of stress. I call this the one-with-nature method, or OWN method. You can adopt this method, when you practice tai chi, and make it your own to achieve self-healing and self-control. The results can be startling.

Lynne, a personnel manager, who complained of a "throbbing stress headache that comes from trying to do too much too fast," comments on the happy results of the 5-minute tai chi headache cure.

"My 9 on a 10-point scale headache went to about a 3. By the end of class, it was almost completely gone. Since the last class, I've had a few more headaches, and each time I've been able to reduce them with the technique you showed me. How wonderful it is to be able to have some control over what has been a rather chronic reaction to stress over the years. Thanks so much."

Cheryl, a young physician, had hurt her right shoulder while playing tennis.

"Dr. Lee had me touch the area with the palm of my left hand, and suggested I use a circular motion, then move my hand down my right arm to the fingertips. After about 5 minutes of this, my soreness was better.

"After this healing session, I completed my 1-hour tai chi lesson, and to my surprise, the pain resolved! Seeing is believing!"

John, a bike racer, who had injured both knees from a fall, healed them using the same method.

"I use tai chi as a way to focus before long races. Usually, I practice three or four times a week. In the weeks immediately before a race, to help me center, I practice daily, often going through the complete sequence twice. The night before the race, I'll practice once or twice in the motel parking lot.

"In October last year, I won the Furnace Creek 508. This is a 512-mile race from Valencia through Death Valley to 29 Palms in the Mojave Desert [California]. I won in 32 hours, becoming the only two-time winner."

The first time John won this race was before his knee injuries. In 1995, he set a course record for an 850-mile race from Reno to Tucson in 54 hours, breaking the old record by 18 hours.

These success stories are typical for Emily's and my tai chi students. In *Ride the Tiger to the Mountain: T'ai Chi for Health* (1989), Emily (Lee), JoAn Johnstone, and I introduced a systematic approach to wellness and the self. We define *self* as a system composed of four elements—mind, body, ch'i, and thought—and *wellness* as composed of four other elements—healing, happiness, health, and harmony.

In this sequel to our first book, Emily and I, and our daughters, Melinda and Joyce, who have practiced tai chi since age 5, describe our personal experiences with self-healing, inner happiness, self-control, and self-realization as well as health and harmony. I hope you can achieve the same benefits as our students. More and more books have illuminated the healing connection between mind and body. To understand this healing process, however, it is essential for us to feel the important connections between mind, body, thought, and ch'i (inner energy).

As you practice the one-with-nature method we describe in this book, you'll be able to understand the relationship between nature and self. You'll be able to reduce and prevent stress in a simple, practical way that heals the mind and body while restoring self-control, something essential to maintaining mastery of both. Stress can be a prime cause of many physical and mental illnesses in modern life. And the relationship between mental and physical stress and the healing process cannot be understood through the study of medicine alone. We need to integrate all our knowledge in science, philosophy, psychology, medicine, physical exercise, and more into a single system that everyone can easily learn. I believe we have taken the first step in this direction.

Writing this book has been an inner journey for us. I hope that my experiences inspire you to have your own one-with-nature journey. As more people take this journey, we will be able to prevent stress, regain control of our lives, and enjoy to the fullest what life has to offer. Our world will be a healthier and more harmonious place when more people become one with nature as Lao Tze describes it: "There exists something which is prior to all beginnings and endings, which, unmoved and unmanifested, itself neither begins nor ends. All pervasive and inexhaustible, it is the perpetual source of everything else. For want of a better name, I call it nature."

Martin Lee, Ph.D.

# One-with-Nature Theory

*"Nature can never be completely described, for such a description of nature would have to duplicate nature. No name can fully express what it represents. It is nature itself, and not any part abstracted from nature, which is the ultimate source of all that happens, all that comes and goes, begins and ends, is and is not. But to describe nature as the 'ultimate source of all' is still only a description, and such a description is not nature itself. Yet since, in order to speak of it, we must use words, we shall have to describe it as 'the ultimate source of all.' "*

Lao Tze
translated by Archie Bahm

*"Once Chuang Chou dreamt he was a butterfly, a butterfly flitting and fluttering around, happy with himself and doing as he pleased. He didn't know he was Chuang Chou. Suddenly he woke up and there he was, solid and unmistakable, Chuang Chou. But he didn't know if he was Chuang Chou who had dreamt he was a butterfly, or a butterfly dreaming he was Chuang Chou."*

Chuang Chou Tze

## Nature and the Self

Coaxed by curiosity, a trait we consider an intrinsic part of human nature, we make great discoveries and succeed in little, important ways in our daily lives. But most great discoveries do not come easily, especially when dealing with fundamental questions about the self and nature. We continue to debate ancient philosophical questions about the relationship of humans to nature. And we probe these questions with science. Who are we? What is nature? What is our place in nature? Chuang Chou, more than 2,000 years ago, described not just human imagination, but a fleeting perception of the self as integral to nature.

Philosophers, scientists, literary men and women, and other thinkers have provided diverse answers to these important questions. But answers to these questions must lie within the mind and heart, where scientific and philosophical modes merge. Scientists make hypotheses to describe physical systems, as Sir Isaac Newton did when describing the motion of a physical force. Consider his hypothesis that for every action there is an equal and opposite reaction.

$$Action = -Reaction$$

This hypothesis allowed Newton to develop classical mechanics, a discipline still used by scientists today to physically describe nature. The word *action* is usually not defined in terms of reactions at all, but it is a definition of action that scientists can use. You, however, might not find it useful in everyday life.

If we are to understand, in a scientific way, the relationship between nature and the self, we must also begin with a hypothesis. For me, as an engineering physicist, nature is a physical system composed of matter and energy. We can call the matter constituting nature the "universe," or the "body of nature." And we can call the physical energies in nature "nature's energy." With these simple terms, we can describe nature in this equation.

Nature = the Universe + All Physical Energies

*or*

Nature = Nature's Body + Nature's Energy

We can use a similar equation to describe nature philosophically. We can begin with a hypothesis based on the assumption that nature is composed of an infinite mind (nature's mind) and an eternal thought (nature's thought). So, we can describe nature in these terms.

Nature = Infinite Mind + Eternal Thought

*or*

Nature = Nature's Mind + Nature's Thought

Some people have described God in similar terms; one dictionary defines *God* as "infinite mind," "eternal," "that which is without beginning and end." *Eternal thought,* then, is thought which has no beginning and no end. For simplicity, we can refer to these attributes as nature's mind and nature's thought.

If we combine these scientific and philosophical approaches to describing nature into one, here is the resulting definition of nature.

Nature = Nature's Mind + Body + Energy + Thought

The word *nature* in this equation represents a physical–philosophical system composed of four essential elements. Since we are part of this physical–philosophical system, our being has the same composition as nature. Therefore, these same four elements may describe ourselves.

Self = Our Mind + Body + Energy + Thought

Note the distinction between thought and the mind. This is because thoughts may be considered things existing within the mind. The mind, in other words, acts as the thoughts' body just as the brain acts as the mind's body. Also, remember that the word *ch'i* means "inner energy," or energy inside the body.

These diagrams illustrate the four elements of each system.

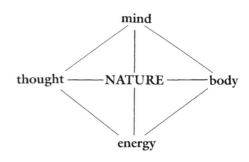

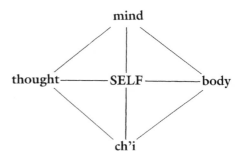

## The Tao of Becoming One with Nature

Let's use the four basic elements of nature and the self to describe the four conditions of being one with nature.

I am one with nature . . .
when my mind is with nature's mind
when my body is with nature's body
when my ch'i is with nature's energy
when my thought is with nature's thought

The four elements of being one with nature can be understood in the diagram on p. 19 in which the self, one's own existence, is surrounded by nature, expressed as universal, infinite, and eternal.

Bringing our state of being in line with that of nature is necessary if we are to make use of nature to heal ourselves. We can begin the process by asking ourselves these four basic questions.

How can my mind be with nature's mind?
How can my body be with nature's body?
How can my ch'i be with nature's energy?
How can my thought be with nature's thought?

We can answer these questions in a simple way by recognizing that since nature created us, nature can also help us become one with itself. In accord with nature, the one-with-nature method described in this book can facilitate this process. Consider the words of Lao Tze.

"Things which act naturally do not need to be told how to act. The wind and rain begin without being ordered and quit without being commanded. This is the way with all natural beginnings and endings. If nature does not have to instruct the wind and rain, how much less should humans try to direct them? Whoever acts naturally is nature itself acting."

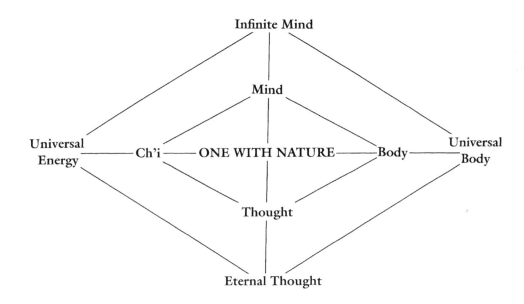

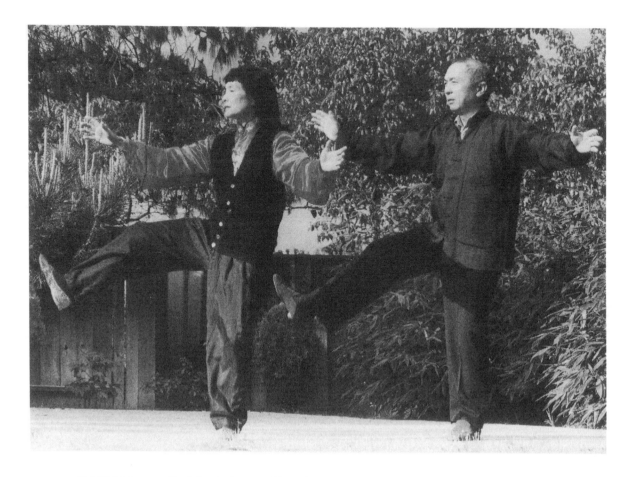

Tai Chi Masters Dr. Martin Lee and Emily Lee (shown above) received a grant from the National Institute of Aging to conduct a study from 1999 to 2002 on the benefits of tai chi for seniors under the Wellness Intervention for Self-Enrichment (WISE) project in association with the Stanford Center for Research on Disease Prevention.

The participants, most of whom were in their mid-70s, were volunteers over age 65. Before the study began, all seniors were in good general health, able to walk without assistance, and classed as "sedentary" because they exercised less than 60 minutes a week.

In this study, the Lees gave the seniors free tai chi instruction.

Study participants practiced tai chi twice a week for 6 months, then once a week for 6 months. The sedentary seniors found many of the same benefits as younger tai chi students. Most seniors were able to incorporate tai chi principles and practice into their daily lives almost immediately. In fact, these seniors, the Lees found, have achieved the same benefits as more active senior students enrolled in their regular Tai Chi for Total Fitness classes.

# CHAPTER TWO

# Becoming One with Nature

Drawing on more than 20 years' experience of teaching tai chi to thousands of students, I devised a simple, practical way of teaching my students how to become one with nature. I often tell beginning students:

"I am a scientist. As a scientist I work with physical systems. But I am also a tai chi master, and as a tai chi master, I also understand the body as a mental and physical system. Let's see what we have inside this mental and physical system: We all have a mind and a body, and inside the mind, we have thoughts. Thoughts are like the coffee inside a cup. The cup, then, is the mind and the coffee represents the thoughts. Similarly, inside the body, we have energy. Because this energy is inside us, we may think of it as *inner energy*."

We are all familiar with the concept of energy. Sunlight outside is, for example, full of energy. Scientists learn about energy by looking outward at nature, and many neglect attending to the energy that exists inside the body. Since nature does not distinguish between outside and inside, energy that exists outside the body must also exist inside. So, the ch'i inside us is the same as the energy to be found outside the body.

In the diagram of the self, four parts—mind, body, ch'i, and thought—are connected and form a single system. Well-being can be defined in terms of the relationships among these four parts. If all these relationships are intact, you are healthy, but if any relationship is not intact, you may get sick. What disrupts the vital, natural relationship of mind, body, ch'i, and thought can trigger loss of good health. Many people today recognize stress as a principal cause of illness.

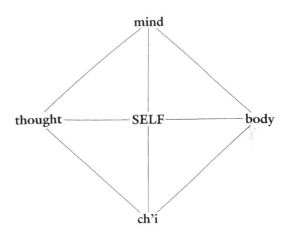

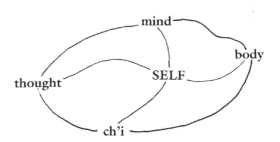

## Happiness and the Mind–Thought Connection

How does stress really affect us? Here is an example of a stressful event everyone will find familiar. Suppose a friend tells you something that bothers you, and you keep repeating the words in your mind. The unpleasant thought may keep you awake at night and you may continue to ponder it the following day. Now it is your own

21

thoughts that bother you as you try to make sense of what your friend said and to discover why he said what he did. For your own sense of well-being, you must find a way to rid your mind of these stress-producing thoughts. This may sound easier than it really is. Why can't you let go of thoughts that made you unhappy?

At these times, the natural relationship between thought and mind is disturbed. Your initial reaction to the unpleasant statement (being upset) is compounded by distress when you continue to ponder its meaning. The usually tranquil relationship between your mind and its thoughts must be restored. When the mind feels it is under stress, it seems to tighten its grip on unpleasant thoughts. This keeps the unhappy thought from leaving the mind. As long as the troublesome thought remains inside your mind, you'll continue to be bothered by it. This situation can make you unhappy or even sorrowful. How can you save yourself from feeling unhappy? The best solution is to allow nature to restore the natural relationship between your thoughts and your mind. You need to calm or quiet your mind, which will then let go of the disturbing thought. This stress-free state could clearly be considered *happiness*.

## Healing and the Body–Ch'i Connection

If stress can "hold" unhappy thoughts inside the mind, what effect could stress have on the body? As you might expect, when we are under stress, the body tightens. As a result, the ch'i inside is affected and its natural flow is altered. Under this situation, the body won't be "happy" either. Although this may sound simplistic, it is a fairly accurate description of what happens inside the body. Aches and pains are merely cries for help; they are the body's way of signaling that you are under stress.

If you analyze what happens to the body when your ch'i is "stuck," you'll realize that the free flow of ch'i can affect wellness. If stress remains

in your head for a period of time, you may get a headache. If it centers in your back, you may develop a backache. The body's organs, like the kidneys and liver, may also be subject to stress and, therefore, to more serious stress-related illnesses. The natural way to heal the body is to rid it of stress. So, we can define *healing* as a state of the body that is stress-free.

Just as we can depend on nature to rid the mind of unpleasant thoughts, a natural mechanism restores the flow of ch'i in the body and rids it of pain. This method is simple: learn to relax the body inside and out. If you ask a physical therapist about relaxing the body, he will probably advise you to relax your muscles. But you need to relax more than your muscles to restore the free flow of ch'i. Internal organs and systems like the pulmonary, nervous, or gastrointestinal system must be relaxed just like your muscular system. While many exercises help relax muscles, few exercises and methods teach us how to relax the inside of the body and mind. Naturally, relaxing complex organs like the brain or lungs is not as simple as adopting an exercise regimen. But nature can relax the mind and every part of the body as well. To understand the four basic elements of being one with nature, consider this chicken-and-egg story.

## The Chicken and the Egg

In just a few weeks, a chick is created and an egg hatched. The chick that hatched from the egg was not made by the hen and rooster alone. The chick is the work of nature. What does a hen have to do to ensure the birth of her chicks? Just four things: relax, breathe, feel the earth beneath her, and then do nothing extra. These actions prevent stress that could adversely affect her unhatched eggs. If the hen feels stress, she may not be able to stay warm, and then her eggs may not hatch. If the hen does something extra, there will not be any chicks. For example, during the hatching process, the hen often gets up and turns the eggs over. Doing nothing extra means she does nothing unnecessary. She does not jump up and down on the eggs, poke holes to see if they are ready to hatch, or take 10-minute breaks. She simply instinctively turns them over.

Chickens, like most creatures in nature, learn how to live without any coaching. They know how to relax, breathe, feel the ground, and do nothing extra. These four basic stress-prevention techniques we all instinctively knew as children. We all naturally know how to relax, breathe, feel the earth, and do nothing extra. Since we all know how to do these four things, we all know how to prevent stress.

An egg, an apparently simple thing, can develop in just a few weeks into a complicated baby chick. If nature can transform an egg into a chicken, surely there's nothing too complicated for nature to do. Relaxing the mind and body are simple tasks if you allow nature to do these things for you. Nature removes stress as soon as the mind and body are back in a state of relaxation and calm. With stress gone, happiness can be restored and healing can take place, naturally and rapidly.

Anyone can become one with nature by doing what the hen does: relaxing, breathing, feeling the earth, and doing nothing extra. Beginning students often find doing nothing extra the most difficult of these four elements. It simply means carry out each task as naturally and instinctively as you can, allowing nature to meet you halfway. The less you do, the more nature will do for you.

## The Four One-with-Nature Elements

I developed these four one-with-nature elements from studying ch'i kung under Dr. Yu Pen-Shih, a distinguished German-educated physician and ch'i kung master from Shanghai, China. During a ch'i kung practice session a student accidentally dislocated his knee. Dr. Yu calmly relocated the knee and then touched the wounded area with his palm. After a few minutes, Dr. Yu asked the student to stand up to see how he felt. At first the student was afraid to stand, worried that he might again dislocate the knee. When he finally gathered enough courage to stand up, the student smiled broadly and shouted, "I feel no pain at all. This is incredible!"

The student later told me he had dislocated his knee before. On other occasions his knee was painful and swollen for weeks.

I had been experiencing joint pain in my right hand, which I had injured a few months earlier while landscaping. I asked Dr. Yu to help me heal the joints, all except one. This way, I could evaluate the results by comparing the healed finger joints with the single finger that remained untreated. Dr. Yu accepted.

When he finished healing my joints, Dr. Yu asked me to move my fingers to see how they felt. To my surprise, I felt no pain in the fingers he had healed, but the unhealed finger remained as painful as before. I could not believe that nearly all pain in my injured hand had gone away in less than 15 minutes.

Later I decided to repeat the experiment to see if I could heal the one finger still in pain. I tried to copy Dr. Yu's method and I tried rubbing and massaging it. But nothing worked, no matter how hard I tried.

A week later, I told Dr. Yu that I had tried to heal myself with no success. He was very patient and explained to me that before I could heal myself, I had to be able to feel ch'i. He also told me about tone ch'i, a traditional method ch'i kung masters use to help students feel ch'i. In Chinese *tone* means "to establish a link or connection," and *tone ch'i* means "to establish a connection between thought and ch'i." After his explanation, Dr. Yu helped me heal my last hurt finger. This time, it took only a few minutes.

**Relax**
**Breathe**
**Feel the Earth**
**Do Nothing Extra**

## Tone Ch'i and the Thought–Ch'i Connection

Months later Dr. Yu helped me learn how to feel ch'i by performing tone ch'i. Before he began, Dr. Yu asked me to assume a ch'i kung stance. Then he placed both palms above my head and told me to relax my entire body and breathe naturally. As I relaxed, I felt a warm and comfortable sensation inside my body moving gently down to the soles of my feet. I call this warm sensation the *inner breath*. When the warm sensation reached my feet, the tone ch'i process, which took about 15 minutes, was complete.

I understood that it was a great honor for a student to be given tone ch'i by a master. This experience with tone ch'i helped me realize the important relationship between ch'i and thought and that this connection could not be made until you are completely relaxed and breathing naturally. I also realized that the warm sensation I felt during the tone ch'i process was the effect of thought and ch'i and that the thought–ch'i connection plays an important role in self-healing.

We can describe the thought–ch'i connection by the energy–mass connection of Einstein's famous equation: $E = mc^2$. Remember, $E$ is energy, $m$ mass, and $c$ the velocity of light. Einstein used this equation to describe the relation of energy and mass in the physical universe. In your own physical and mental universe, a similar connection exists between thought and ch'i. Understanding the thought–ch'i connection provides a key to the mystery of ch'i.

## Inner Breath and Inner Happiness

After learning how to feel my inner breath during tone ch'i, I tried to recreate this experience when I practiced ch'i kung, tai chi, and meditation. By doing this, I found a simple way to feel the inner breath by relaxing my entire body, using my whole body to breathe, feeling the earth beneath me, and making sure I was doing nothing extra.

I was able to achieve the same warm sensation and good feeling no matter what practice I engaged in. The good feeling coming from inside I call *inner happiness*. Both inner happiness and the flow of the inner breath come from the relaxation process brought from the connection of my thought and ch'i.

I also found that you can enhance this warm, good feeling of inner happiness and inner breath during exhalation. Exhalation is a voluntary action in which the outward flow of air creates a vacuum in the lungs. Inhalation, however, is a natural response in which air is sucked into the lungs naturally by this vacuum. As air is exhaled through your mouth, you can feel the inner breath moving to different parts of your body. With practice, you can feel and direct this flow of inner breath by thinking and breathing. The whole mind-and-body relaxation process involves the *intention* to relax, breathe, feel the earth, and do nothing extra, and *attention* to these things.

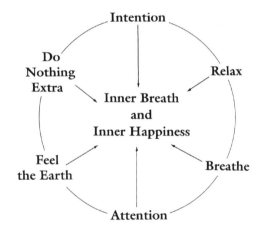

Relaxation, for me, means relaxing every part of the body, including internal organs like the kidneys and the lungs as well as blood vessels and nerves. The only way to do this is by using the mind and body's connection to thought and ch'i. The word *breathe* here means breathing with every part of the body, which you can achieve through the thought–ch'i connection. This also applies to "feel the earth" and "do nothing extra." When you practice these four elements, you will find that relaxing, breathing, feeling the earth, and doing nothing extra are interdependent.

> To *relax* completely, breathe, feel the earth, and do nothing extra with your whole body.
> To *breathe* fully, relax, feel the earth, and do nothing extra with your whole body.
> To *feel the earth* fully, relax, breathe, and do nothing extra with your whole body.
> To *do nothing extra*, relax, breathe, and feel the earth with your whole body.

Through the thought–ch'i connection you can practice these four one-with-nature elements at the same time.

Practicing these four elements together will help you become one with nature. These four one-with-nature elements can be expressed with this formula.

OWN Elements = Relax + Breathe + Feel the Earth + Do Nothing Extra

## The Thought–Ch'i Connection and the One-with-Nature Method

The thought–ch'i connection allows you to use thinking and breathing to relax your entire body and your mind. Many people consider breathing a fact of life, since everybody knows how to breathe. When you hold your breath, the body tenses up and creates more stress within, without your even knowing it. So, the thought–ch'i connection plays an essential role in stress reduction as well as prevention of stress.

We often create stress within ourselves when we are angry, when we hurry, when we feel sadness or sorrow, and when we worry. Everybody knows how difficult it is to control the mind and body when we experience these emotions. Unless we are able to prevent these painful experiences, the body and mind will come under stress which may lead to loss of happiness, health, harmony, and the body and mind's ability to heal themselves.

Several methods can help you learn the thought–ch'i connection. Although all these methods allow you to achieve the goal of becoming one with nature, each method also brings special benefits that ultimately can help you regain healing, happiness, health, and harmony. You'll learn about these one-with-nature methods and their benefits in the next chapters.

# CHAPTER THREE

# One-with-Nature Tone Ch'i and Inner Happiness

*"Happiness is the very nature of the self; happiness and the self are not different."*
*Bhagavan Sri Ramana Maharishi*

## Inner Happiness

We spend much energy on everyday emotions, which we take great pains to analyze. Consider happiness. For most people, happiness is just a state of mind. But there's another kind of happiness, a natural state of the self which occurs when stress is removed from both the body and the mind. It includes mind, body, ch'i, and thought; it is not just a state of the mind alone.

## One-with-Nature Tone Ch'i

The four one-with-nature elements, combined with Grand Tai Chi (see p. 139), can help you feel your inner breath and regain inner happiness. This combination can be called the *One-with-Nature Tone Ch'i*.

One-with-Nature Tone Ch'i = Four One-with-Nature Elements + Grand Tai Chi

I have used the tone-ch'i movement for more than 20 years to introduce the practice of becoming one with nature to beginning students. I chose the Grand Tai Chi movement because it allows students to calm the mind and relax the whole body. As students become one with nature, the tone-ch'i movement helps them reduce stress and feel good, inside and outside, physically and mentally. This movement is an efficient method to gain happiness, defined as a balanced, stress-free natural state.

## Learning One-with-Nature Tone Ch'i

Get ready for the tone-ch'i movement by practicing the four one-with-nature elements: relax, breathe, feel the earth, and do nothing extra, one at a time. Review the "get ready" position on the opposite page. Then learn to combine these four one-with-nature elements with Grand Tai Chi, a movement that may also be considered an independent form (see p. 139), to create One-with-Nature Tone Ch'i. For practicing One-with-Nature Tone Ch'i, refer to the photo and instructions for steps *a* to *d*, and observe the drawings for the get-ready and end positions (all on p. 27, opposite).

By practicing this One-with-Nature Tone Ch'i a few times, you will be able to feel relaxed and calm if you pay attention to the inside of your body as you lower your arms. As a beginner, you may experience this relaxed and calm feeling only in the upper part of your body. However, with practice, you will be able to feel a wonderful and soothing sensation that reaches down to your feet. When you feel this inner happiness, you will become one with nature. When the body and mind are under stress, we often cannot feel this happiness. However, when you relax, breathe, feel the earth, perform this movement, and do

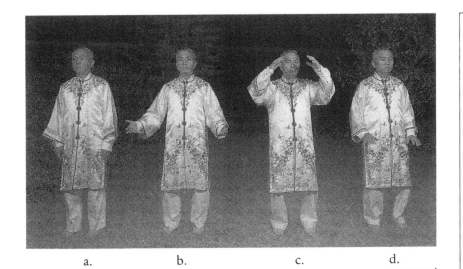
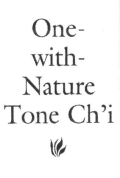

a.    b.    c.    d.

## One-with-Nature Tone Ch'i

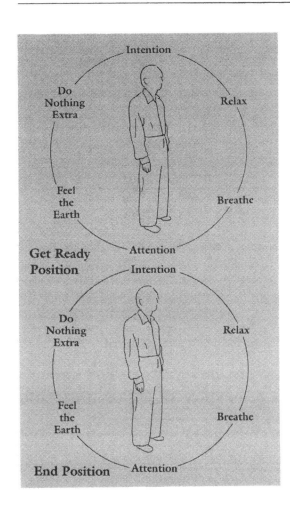

**Get Ready Position**

Intention · Relax · Breathe · Attention · Feel the Earth · Do Nothing Extra

**End Position**

Intention · Relax · Breathe · Attention · Feel the Earth · Do Nothing Extra

### Get Ready Position

**Relax**   Stand with your feet parallel with arms at your sides and relax your whole body by thinking and feeling.

**Breathe**   As the body relaxes, breathe smoothly and naturally.

**Feel the Earth**   So that the whole body feels connected with the ground, bend the knees slightly and evenly. Feel the body's weight on the feet.

**Do Nothing Extra**   See that you are relaxing, breathing, and feeling the earth naturally.

### One-with-Nature Tone Ch'i

**a.** Assume the "get ready position" (relax, breathe, feel the earth, and do nothing extra).

**b.** Bend the knees evenly, turn the palms out, and raise your hands slowly to temple height. Continue to relax, breathe, feel the earth, and do nothing extra.

**c.** Turn the palms down and close the eyes. Relax, breathe, feel the earth, and do nothing extra.

**d.** Lower the hands down to the sides slowly and evenly. Relax, breathe, feel the earth, and do nothing extra.

nothing extra, you'll be able to release stress from the body and the mind and experience inner happiness.

Inner breath and inner happiness are natural responses to tone-ch'i movement, when your thought and ch'i combine with nature's thought and nature's ch'i. Since the mind, body, ch'i, and

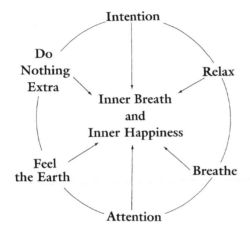

thought are linked and since your thought is with nature's thought and your ch'i with nature's ch'i, tone-ch'i movement enables your mind to be with nature's mind and your body to be with nature's body. Practicing tone-ch'i movement is the fastest way to achieve the state of being one with nature. That's because inner happiness comes naturally from within, due to the thought–ch'i connection.

One-with-Nature Movement → Thought–Ch'i Connection → Inner Happiness

# How Tone Ch'i Works

Observing how well tone ch'i could make one feel one with nature, I asked myself how it worked. So, I studied what happened when I practiced the movement. I like to think about this inner process the way I think about linear accelerators.

## Problem and Solution for an Accelerator

An accelerator has two parts: the machine and a particle beam. At Stanford University, for example, we have an accelerator consisting of a two-mile wave-guide structure that looks like a pipe with thousands of discs inside. Outside this pipe are a few hundred magnets. The beam is a bunch of electrons, about 10 billion. The idea is to shoot an electron bunch down the machine along the axis of the pipe. In an ideal machine, when all magnets are centered properly around the pipe, the beam will travel along the axis naturally and uninterrupted. However, if the magnets are off-center, then the beam is deflected from the axis and it will fail to deliver a useful beam at the end of the machine.

To solve this problem, we first have to know where the beam is along the machine at any given time. We do this by using sensors to measure the beam's position as it passes through the pipe. Then, we must position the magnets one at a time until the beam is not deflected as it passes through each magnet along the axis. In a way, we use the beam itself to tell us what we have to do to make it pass through the accelerator properly.

## Problem and Solution for the Self

Think of the body as a system not unlike an accelerator. Suppose, for instance, that your body is composed of a stack of one-inch sections called "subselves." Here each subself can be described by the same four elements as the whole self.

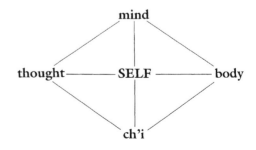

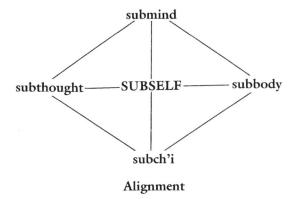

**Alignment**

The four subself elements are like the four poles of a quadrupole magnet in an accelerator section. The inner breath is like an electron beam. What happens when the self comes under stress? Some of the subselves also feel stress. As a result, the submind, subbody, subch'i, and subthought may become misaligned just as magnets do in an accelerator. As the inner breath passes through a misaligned subself, it will be deflected just like the beam when a magnet is misaligned. Instead of passing from one section of the body to the next, the inner breath becomes stuck in the particular section that is under stress. It is deflected in that section and cannot continue on its path.

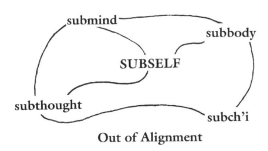

**Out of Alignment**

To resolve this problem, first you need to actually feel the inner breath as it passes along the body by feeling the warm sensation as you exhale. When you find the part of the body where you don't feel the inner breath, you can relax it by using your thought and ch'i. You can repeat this procedure as often as necessary until you can feel the inner breath reaching all the way to your feet.

I call this procedure inner breath self-realignment, because as it passes through the body, you can use the inner breath itself to tell you what to do, just as the particle beam tells the operator of a linear accelerator when one of the magnets is out of alignment.

One-with Nature Tone Ch'i works so well because as you lower your hands inch by inch, you can feel your inner breath move down inch by inch and remove stress from your body and mind also inch by inch. As you feel the inner breath down to your feet, your whole self becomes realigned with nature. Inner happiness here is the happy-with-myself feeling that comes naturally from this realignment.

I've taught the tone-ch'i movement to many groups, including younger children. I gave a talk on stress reduction at a high school for students with learning problems. I asked, with the aid of a physician, Margaret, two questions: (1) How did you feel before doing the movement? (2) How did you feel after doing the movement? The students ranked themselves on a scale from 1 to 10, with 1 indicating completely calm and 10 completely tense. Seven of the nine students said they felt calmer after the tone-ch'i movement, and four students reported substantial benefits from the tone-ch'i movement (going from 10 to 1, 10 to 2, 10 to 5, and 7 to 3, the first number before and the second after the movement).

A first-grade teacher, Carlo, who taught his students the tone-ch'i movement, reported these results.

"I have a very bad group of first-graders this year. About half of them are hyperactive kids. You should see what they did in the first few days of this semester. In the morning, they were all over the classroom—running, screaming, chasing each other, shouting loudly, and even kicking each other. I tried the normal way of dealing with them with no success. Then, I taught them the tone-ch'i movement. It calmed most of them down—except a couple of real super-active ones. Because they love it, I am now doing it every morning."

## Inner Happiness for Everybody

I'm very thankful Dr. Yu taught me the importance of inner happiness and helped me experience tone ch'i. My students have demonstrated that inner happiness can be self-taught. The tone-ch'i movement produces the same feelings as tone ch'i without outside help.

After a few times practicing this movement, you will be able to experience the wonderful feeling of being one with nature. With this tone-ch'i movement, you can experience inner happiness more quickly. And if people feel happy about themselves, perhaps humanity will begin to feel happier and the world will become a more pleasant place. If you have only 30 seconds to make yourself feel better, you can do the tone-ch'i movement. And you can put Lao Tze's philosophy into practice: "He who receives his happiness from others may be rich, but he whose contentment is self-willed has inexhaustible wealth."

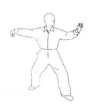

# CHAPTER FOUR

# One-with-Nature Tai Chi and Self-Control

*"To move, move every part. To be still, quiet every part."*                    *Tai Chi Proverb*

*"He who controls others may be powerful, but he who has mastered himself is mightier still."*
                                              *Tao Te Ching*
                              translated by Archie Bahm

*"If you could stand grounded at the age of 30, hold your thought steady at 40, control your action at 50, and not be disturbed by what you hear at 60, then you will know your own destiny by the time you are 70."*
                                              *Confucius*

## Self-Control

Self-control, though not usually thought of as a recipe for health and harmony, plays an important part in maintaining a good, happy life. Being in control does not mean behaving like an automaton, living by strict rules, do's and don't's. It merely helps us maintain good thoughts while freeing us from unnecessary distress. Self-control simply means that if you want to be happy, let go of unhappy thoughts. If you want to avoid stress-induced pain, you must learn how to prevent stress from building up inside the body. Since both healing and happiness depend on control of your actions toward yourself, you must learn to control not only your mind and body but also your thoughts and ch'i. Here's a definition of self-control.

Self-Control = Control of Mind + Body + Ch'i + Thought

## Accelerator Control and Self-Control

The operation of a physical plant like a linear accelerator depends on its control system, which must be able to perform multiple tasks. The more tasks it can perform, the better the system. This situation is also true for the "control" of a personality. And we can argue that the more tasks a person can perform well, the more control that person effectively has over himself.

Consider artificial intelligence, the use of computers and machines to control a complex physical plant. With the use of artificial intelligence, a control system is actually able to adapt itself to situations by learning with a training set of events. Artificial intelligence, such as neural networks, involves first training the control system, then controlling the plant automatically.

One-with-nature tai chi can function like a training set with its 64 movements. And each movement in turn involves five tasks, the four one-with-nature elements plus the physical movement. Every movement begins as a mental intention, determining what to do, that's guided by both thinking and feeling. Through the power of the one-with-nature elements—relax, breathe, feel the earth, and do nothing extra—the flow of the inner breath naturally responds to this mental intention. By paying attention to exhalation, you can feel the inner breath moving toward different parts of the body. The practice of one-with-nature tai chi will enable you to gain control of your mind, body, thought, and ch'i at the same time. With these four under control, you'll be able to relax, breathe, feel the earth, and do nothing extra whenever you need to become one with nature. And you'll be able to prevent yourself from feeling stress in everyday life.

In addition, these 64 movements are not just a training set that allows you to gain control of your mind, body, ch'i, and thought naturally, but they are also exercises that promote good health. As a natural response to the flow of the inner breath and the feeling of inner happiness, stress is released. The release of stress also brings happiness and healing to every part of the body naturally.

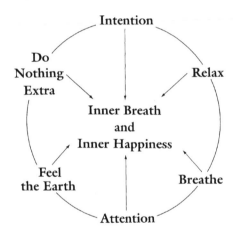

## Learning One-with-Nature Tai Chi

To begin learning a particular movement, first learn the starting and the end positions. Then, practice the movement by moving from the starting to the end position in the most natural way. As you move from one position to the next, keep in mind the need to relax, breathe, feel the earth, and do nothing extra.

For example, to learn the first tai-chi form, Pay Respect to Buddha (Humankind), learn the start-ing and end positions by looking at the drawings that accompany the description of the movement (see p. 62). After you are able to relax, breathe, feel the earth, and do nothing extra in these two positions, learn the first movement by following the written directions while looking at the photo. After you have learned a new form, add it to the ones you have already learned and practice them together, one after another. To complete a sequence, end your practice with the form Grand Tai Chi (see p. 139), which combines one-with-nature elements with the tone-ch'i movement (see pp. 26–27). See the list of names of forms and relative body orientation for each on pp. 55–59.

## The Thought–Ch'i Connection

Since tai chi was originally developed as a boxing routine, every form (this book includes 64 forms) involves a self-defense action with the arm or leg, like pulling, pushing, punching, deflecting, or kicking. Performing the movements with the correct intention and attention, you will be able to connect your thinking with your body's movement.

Begin each movement of each form with an intention of what you will be doing. Your intention not only controls and coordinates each movement, but it has the power of being able to direct ch'i into every part of the body. The slow timing of tai chi forms allows this guiding intention to precede each movement. While you are performing the movement, pay attention to how you are doing it. Relax, breathe, feel the earth, and do nothing extra as you attend to how you feel inside. Gradually, your breathing and the flow of ch'i will be naturally regulated by your movement.

For beginners, achieving self-control and practicing one-with-nature elements with tai chi may appear complicated. As you relax, breathe, feel the earth, do nothing extra, and perform the 64 forms through connecting your thought with your ch'i, you gain self-control quite naturally.

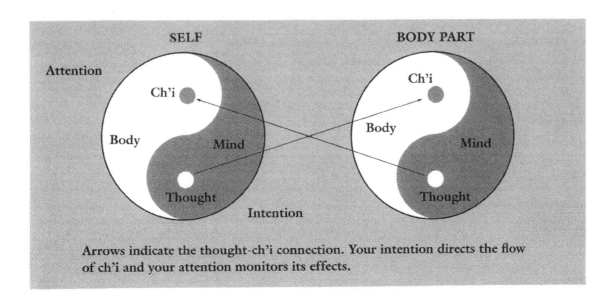

**Arrows indicate the thought-ch'i connection. Your intention directs the flow of ch'i and your attention monitors its effects.**

One-with-Nature Tai Chi → Thought–Ch'i Connection → Self-Control

For example, when you practice the first form with an intention to block with your left arm while attending to how the weight on your right leg feels, this Pay Respect to Buddha (Humankind) form will enhance the thought–ch'i connection between your left arm and right leg.

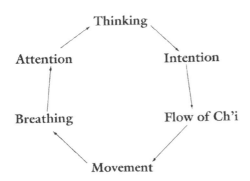

**Arrows indicate the process of thinking and moving. The right side of the circle shows how intention guides movement, and the left side shows how attention monitors effects of the movements.**

## Benefits from Gaining Self-Control

From over 20 years of teaching one-with-nature tai chi, we find that most students develop some degree of self-control after learning the first twelve tai chi forms. As students gain more self-control, we also notice an improved ability to achieve inner happiness. Some students can feel the inner breath flowing to different parts of the body during their first few weeks of classes. After they practice one-with-nature tai chi for a while, they begin to understand the meaning of the four elements. Every part of the body can relax, breathe, feel the earth, and do nothing extra at the same time. When students incorporate these four elements into their daily activities, they will be able to do everything better and to enjoy these activities more.

Jerry, an electrician, had lost his job because of a serious back injury.

"After treatment for a year and a half, doctors said nothing else could be done except to fuse five discs and install two rods in my spine. That's when I changed doctors. My new physician . . . thought a plan of physical therapy and treatment with injections and medications would prove to be a better course of action. . . .

33

"My recovery now is nothing less than miraculous. With the help of Martin and Emily Lee, I have been able to regain a part of my life which I thought was gone forever. Because of the nature of my injury, I had been confined to the home for most of the last three years. But now I am able to again do things that I once took for granted. I have been able to regain mobility. I can now drive short distances in the car, and the general feeling of well-being and health is mine every day, instead of the constant pain and anxiety that I have had to go through. . . . I attribute my improved mental and physical condition completely to the practice of tai chi. . . ."

John, an associate dean at Stanford University, explains what he gained from practicing tai chi and the one-with-nature elements.

"I started tai chi in the fall, 1992. I still remember the first session where you simply had us stand on one leg with knees slightly bent. After a couple of minutes, my big quads and tough biker legs were trembling while you stood calm and relaxed. I learned something that night about different kinds of strength.

"In February, 1993, I was called to Oregon, where my mother was critically ill. I spent three weeks in residence at the hospital. Each morning I would practice tai chi on the roof as a way of calming my emotions and gathering strength for the day ahead before going down to the intensive care unit. . . . I learned what a powerful discipline tai chi is under stressful conditions."

After winning a bike race from California to Arizona, John experimented with tai chi while riding his bike. Remember, being able to do several tasks at the same time is a sign of self-control. He developed his own version of the one-with-nature elements.

"To race long distances, I need to stay focused, not waste energy, and be comfortable on the bike for long periods. A win is not the result of strength and speed, but the ability to keep up a consistent pace and stay on the bike for a long time. Here are some of the ways I use tai chi while riding.

*Relax, Breathe, and Feel the Pedals.*—A simple way of focusing and making sure that my legs are loose and spinning rather than tight and pounding. If I am riding really well, my legs will actually feel like a waterwheel, turned by a constant flow of energy (ch'i).

*Do Nothing Extra.*—I try to keep a relaxed style, not bobbing my head or rocking my shoulders as I pedal. I also try to maintain a constant level of effort, not wasting energy on needless spurts forward.

"After I have been on the bike 8 or 9 hours, my back, shoulders, and neck start to get stiff. If I am on a quiet road with no traffic hazards, I will spend some time imagining that I am doing tai chi, especially parts like Wave Hands Like Clouds (one of the forms). I try to imagine the movement and then feel the same relaxation in my upper body.

"After a long climb, when my legs are very tired and full of lactic acid, I will descend with 'a solid leg and a hollow leg' (a basic way to move in tai chi): The foot of the solid leg is down at 12 o'clock, but with the knee flexed slightly. The foot of the hollow leg is up at 6 o'clock. I try to relax both legs and feel the energy (ch'i) flowing. The relaxation helps the blood move these waste products out."

John's story clearly demonstrates the benefit of practicing one-with-nature elements while bicycling. You can benefit more from any exercise you choose if you relax, breathe, feel the earth, and do nothing extra while you move your body. And here's how you can practice being one-with-nature while standing or walking.

## Walking or Standing

Learn how to practice being one-with-nature when you're in a standing position and when you're walking.

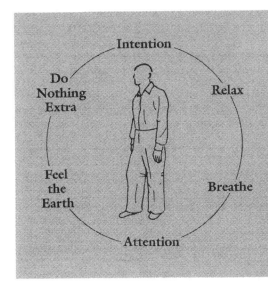

**One-with-Nature Standing or Walking**

1. Stand with feet parallel and the knees slightly bent.
2. Turn one foot slightly outward and shift your weight to this leg.
3. Relax, breathe, feel the earth, and do nothing extra.
4. Move the other foot slightly forward.
5. Repeat, reversing the positions of your legs.

*Intention and Attention:* Relax, breathe, feel the earth, and do nothing extra.

If you practice One-with-Nature Standing or Walking, you will be able to strengthen your legs naturally after a few weeks. And you will no longer have tired legs at the end of the day. If you walk with knees slightly bent while you relax, breathe, feel the earth, and do nothing extra, you will be able to walk longer distances and enjoy walking more. If you always stand and walk this one-with-nature way, you will not put stress on your back. So, this is also a natural way to prevent backaches.

# CHAPTER FIVE

# One-with-Nature Meditation and Self-Realization

"Know thyself," the Greek oracle's injunction to the human race, remains as important today as it was over 2,000 years ago. But attaining and acting on self-knowledge is difficult for all of us, at least while we're young.

One-with-nature method used in meditation can help us achieve that understanding. You can also achieve self-realization using one-with-nature meditation. Nature is intelligent, and it shares this intelligence with us when we are in harmony with it. Practicing one-with-nature meditation may give you more than you would expect. Perhaps you'll be able, as some students have, to become more imaginative and intuitive, if you want these things to happen. This desire will also help you find ways to solve personal dilemmas. I believe that answers to our own questions are to be found within the depths of the mind. It's just a matter of discovering them as you search for who you are. Practicing this meditation can help you get there and help you understand the words of Lao Tze, "He who knows much about others may be learned, but he who understands himself is more intelligent."

## One-with-Nature Meditation

When I first practiced meditation, I used to count my breaths as a means of quieting my mind. Eventually, I discovered that I could quiet my mind much more quickly by paying attention to my inner breath and feeling my inner happiness. As your mind becomes quiet in meditation, you will be able to gain control of your mind more and more. Meditation involves thinking nothing ex-

tra, an extension of the do-nothing-extra element integral to the one-with-nature method in this book.

Thinking nothing extra is simply a way to describe the quieting of the mind, but this is one of the most difficult things for beginners to learn. Imagine yourself in a subway station watching trains pass by. Your thoughts are like those trains. As long as you don't get aboard, you are not thinking extra thoughts. If you happen to hop into a "train," you can get off by feeling your inner breath. For beginners, the easiest way to achieve the think-nothing-extra state is by feeling the inner breath. Feeling the inner breath allows you to check to see whether the whole body is relaxed and your breathing is smooth.

There are many different ways to meditate. Although the postures in various meditation practices may appear similar, the method of thinking, breathing, doing, and feeling can be different. One-with-nature meditation combines the four one-with-nature elements and meditation.

One-with-Nature Meditation = Relax + Breathe + Feel the Earth + Do Nothing Extra + Think Nothing Extra

### Learning One-with-Nature Meditation

Remember the importance of the one-with-nature elements. To relax your whole body and mind, find a natural and comfortable position. You may prefer to sit in a chair or on the floor, whichever is more comfortable and less distracting. After you find this position, you will be able to practice the one-with-nature elements more easily. Although meditation is often interpreted as a way to quiet the mind, the process actually involves all four parts of the self—the mind, body, ch'i, and thought. Since the body is not moving, the connection between thought and ch'i is especially enhanced. Probably the easiest way to quiet the mind is through the thought–ch'i connection. Here's how to practice one-with-nature meditation.

## One-with-Nature Benefits

One-with-nature meditation will enable you to calm your mind and relax your body at the same time by unifying your thought and ch'i with nature's thought and nature's ch'i. Because you are not moving your body, you'll be able to feel all the one-with-nature good feelings more strongly throughout the time you meditate. Therefore, benefits to your mind and body are greatly enhanced. As you become one-with-nature, your mind settles down into its natural, uncluttered, unfettered state. Inner happiness can be attained in this state. When you feel your inner breath in every part of your body, you will experience inner happiness, a state that comes from within.

Meditation is yet another way to gain self-control. When you practice tai chi, you also gain self-control by learning how to do nothing extra physically. When you meditate, however, you can gain self-control by learning how to do nothing extra mentally. Because meditation directly involves the mind, it is an effective way to gain control of your

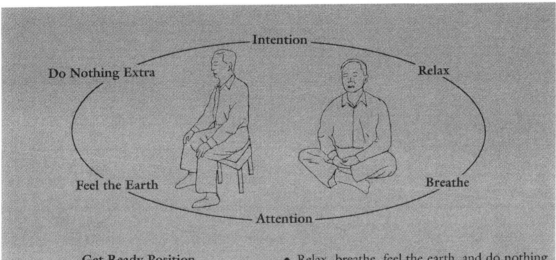

### Get Ready Position

- Sit comfortably on a firm chair with knees bent at a 90° angle. Place your feet parallel a shoulder's width apart, and place your palms gently on your knees. You can also sit comfortably on a cushion or pillow on the floor with legs crossed, and place the left hand on the right palm in front of the abdomen.
- Loosen your back while keeping it straight.
- Relax the face, neck, shoulders, arms, wrists, fingers, legs, ankles, and toes.

- Relax, breathe, feel the earth, and do nothing extra.
- Close the eyes gently to feel the inner breath as you exhale through the mouth.

### One-with-Nature Meditation

- Think nothing extra.
- If a thought appears, practice the four one-with-nature elements and feel the inner breath again.

mind. And with this greater control, you can also gain inner happiness and let go of unpleasant thoughts. By using the inner breath during meditation, you can heal the body at the same time.

Because meditation works directly on the mind and thought, you can even change your temperament, since the state of the mind determines who we are. When I complimented Dr. Yu, ch'i kung master, on his kindness and Buddhalike temperament, he admitted, to my surprise, that he had had a very hot temper in the years before he practiced meditation. He claimed that only Chang Fai, the Chinese general of ancient times whose fury curved his whiskers up all around his face, had as bad a temper. According to a Chinese proverb, "It is harder to change a person's temperament than to move a mountain." But with nature's help, we can accomplish this seemingly impossible task. Besides all these benefits is the additional benefit of self-realization that you can gain with one-with-nature meditation.

## Self-Realization

As children we acquired knowledge by attending school, reading books, doing homework, and interacting with others. By practicing meditation, we can also discover knowledge about ourselves. Self-realization may be achieved by developing one's mental capabilities through the thought–ch'i connection, which allows you to look deep inside yourself. This is the ultimate result of practicing one-with-nature meditation, a state that can be achieved when your mind, body, ch'i, and thought are one with nature's mind, body, ch'i, and thought. In this one-with-nature state, you'll be able to find wisdom from within.

One-with-Nature Meditation → Thought–Ch'i
Connection → Self-Realization

A Zen tale may help you understand how this looking-inward process works.

A young student went with a Zen master to visit the Temple of the Three Monkeys. The master asked, "Who are the three monkeys?" The student looked at the statue of these monkeys and replied, "See No Evil, Hear No Evil, and Speak No Evil." The master said, "Close your eyes and look again." The student was puzzled at first. But it didn't take long before the student responded, "Yes, I see another monkey." As the master asked, "Who is that monkey?", a thought suddenly came into the student's mind. He answered immediately, "Think No Evil."

As this tale suggests, the process of looking from within involves two parts. First, asking yourself a question, and second, actually seeing the answer take shape inside your mind. You can use this two-part process to find answers to personal philosophical questions, such as "Who am I?" and "What's the meaning of life?" When you're in the state of thinking nothing extra, your mind will be at its clearest, and so, it can function at its optimum. In this state of mind, you'll be able to seek knowledge from nature. With this self-realization process, you can put the wisdom of Lao Tze into practice.

"Without going out of doors, one can know all he needs to know. Without even looking out of his window, one can grasp the nature of everything. Without going beyond his own nature, one can achieve ultimate wisdom. Therefore, the intelligent man knows all he needs to know without going away. And sees all he needs to see without looking elsewhere, and does all he needs to do without undue exertion."

# CHAPTER SIX

# One-with-Nature Touch and Self-Healing

## Self-Healing

Using the one-with-nature method, meditation, and tai chi, you've learned in these chapters how to achieve inner happiness, self-control, and self-realization. But many things can interfere with attaining these states. Pain, for instance, not only reduces inner happiness, but it increases the stress you feel in the body and mind, which also affects thought and ch'i. It's difficult to be happy when you are experiencing pain. But most people accept pain as the price of a busy lifestyle, and many take pain-killers like aspirin. However, you can heal yourself in nature's way with a process we call one-with-nature touch, which results in self-healing. Just as the inner breath can produce the feeling of inner happiness, you can use one-with-nature touch to counteract pain located in a specific part of your body.

*Self-healing* involves healing the body by yourself without the aid of any person or medication. If you use this simple method, you'll be able to relieve *stress-induced* pain within minutes and immediately promote the natural healing process. Pain that is not stress-induced is more difficult to deal with and may require medical attention.

The healing power demonstrated from being one with nature is both simple and amazing. When we feel discomfort, we instinctively touch or massage the spot that hurts. If you bump your elbow, for instance, the first thing you do is softly massage your elbow. Usually, when the injury is minor, you feel better right away. But when you combine the same gentle touch with the four one-with-nature elements—relax, breathe, feel the earth, do nothing extra—you'll do more. You can both heal your body and also experience the warm feeling of the inner breath that brings inner happiness.

## One-with-Nature Touch

After trial and error I discovered that I could combine the one-with-nature elements with touch for self-healing.

Four One-with-Nature Elements + Touch = One-with-Nature Touch

The method is simple. If you have a headache, softly touch the area where the pain is with your palm (see illustration). After a few gentle touches, then cover the painful spot with your palm and exhale through your mouth to feel the inner breath between your palm and the painful spot.

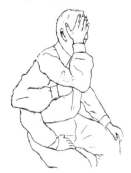

**Self-Healing for a Headache**

Next move your hand down to your chest and then to your leg. While lowering your hand, follow your inner breath as it flows down to your feet. Repeat this healing process until the pain passes, usually within a few minutes.

This self-healing process comes naturally from within because of the thought–ch'i connection. What heals you is not just an external massage, but the inner breath that helps relax a specific body part internally. As the body relaxes, stress can be released from the area, ch'i can flow naturally again, and the pain fades away.

One-with-Nature Touch → Thought–Ch'i Connection → Self-Healing

Since pain is simply a distress signal, if you have no stress at all, then you will not have pain. But stress sometimes returns unannounced, so we need a method to counteract it. One-with-nature touch works because the four elements draw on nature's power to heal through your intention and attention to healing yourself.

## Testing the Self-Healing Method

I tested one-with-nature touch with tai chi students and with people unfamiliar with tai chi. Members of the Stanford University Crew were unfamiliar with ch'i but very familiar with pain and injuries from rowing. Four selected team members who had been injured or who had stress-related pain all felt better after their first lesson in self-healing. Here's what I asked them to do.

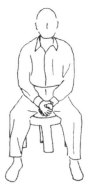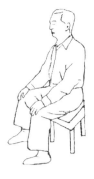

### Self-Healing Preparation

**Feel the inner breath between palms and between palms and knees.**

**40**

### Self-Healing Preparation
- Sit comfortably in a chair.
- Put hands together and move your palms around each other in circles slowly.
- Feel both hands touching each other by paying attention to the place between the palms.
- Exhale a few times through a slightly opened mouth.
- Feel the warm sensation between your palms while exhaling.
- After you feel the warmth, place your palms on your knees as in the sitting meditation position, take a few more breaths gently, and exhale again through your mouth.
- Feel the warm sensation between your palms and knees, and follow this sensation as it travels down to your feet.

After you are able to feel your inner breath, then apply the one-with-nature touch to yourself in the spot where you feel pain.

### One-with-Nature Touch for Self-Healing
1. Relax, breathe, feel the earth (floor), do nothing extra, and touch the painful spot with your palm in a circular motion several times. Cover this spot with your palm, exhale through your mouth, and feel the warm sensation between your palm and the painful spot.
2. Move your palm down slowly over your chest, arm, or leg while exhaling through your mouth.
3. Feel your inner breath flowing down your body, arm, hand, or feet as your palm moves downward.

*Repeat these three steps a few times.*

Although the steps in one-with-nature touch are essentially the same for different types of pain in different locations, you may want to vary specific actions depending on where you feel pain. Here are examples of the rowers and others.

## Healing a Small Area

**Case History**  The coach of the rowing crew had pain in his heel for two years. No conventional treatments seemed to work on the pain, which he described as a 9 on a 10-point scale.

**The Lesson**  I asked the coach to follow my motions as I applied one-with-nature touch to my own heel, using my palm. After 5 minutes, when the coach tried the technique himself, he reported that the pain went down to a 2 and was concentrated in a much smaller area. Since the pain had decreased from a 9 to a 2, I decided that the method was working and the heel pain was induced by stress rather than a more serious condition. Since the pain was reduced to a small spot on his heel, I demonstrated how to touch this area using my finger. As I touched this spot, I felt my inner breath between my finger and the spot. After touching it for a couple of minutes, I repeated the healing touch with my palms.

When the coach followed this healing technique, his pain vanished, to his pleasant surprise. In just 10 minutes, he had relieved two years of excruciating pain. I suggested that he repeat the technique if the pain recurred.

## Healing a Large Area

**Case History**  Mark had two sore thighs. I asked him which leg was more sore and worked on healing that leg, his right. If after the experiment his right leg felt better than his left, we could consider the experiment a success.

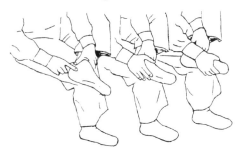

**Self-Healing a Small Area (Heel)**

**The Lesson**  Since Mark's right leg's soreness spread over a large area, I applied the one-with-nature method using both hands. After copying my motions for 5 minutes, Mark said his soreness had been reduced about 40 percent. I continued to apply the feeling–ch'i touch to my right leg and Mark copied my movements. Two minutes later, Mark's pain had disappeared completely from his right leg. A week later Mark applied the same method to his left leg and eliminated the soreness he felt.

## Healing a Hard-to-Reach Area

You can easily touch your feet and legs with your palms, but how do you heal places you cannot reach easily with your palms? Since nature is within and around us, we can apply the one-with-nature touch near the area of pain and heal the pain even when we cannot reach the painful area itself.

**Case History**  John had pain deep in his upper back in an area difficult to reach from behind with his palm.

**The Lesson**  I showed John how to apply the one-with-nature touch on his chest in front of the painful area rather than on the upper back itself. While he was touching his chest, I suggested that he feel his inner breath flowing from front to back. With this modification of one-with-nature touch, John's pain went down to about 20 percent after several minutes. Since nature does not distinguish between the front and back of the body, the method works. John later reported that the pain disappeared the day after this lesson.

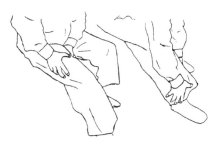

**Self-Healing a Large Area (Thigh)**

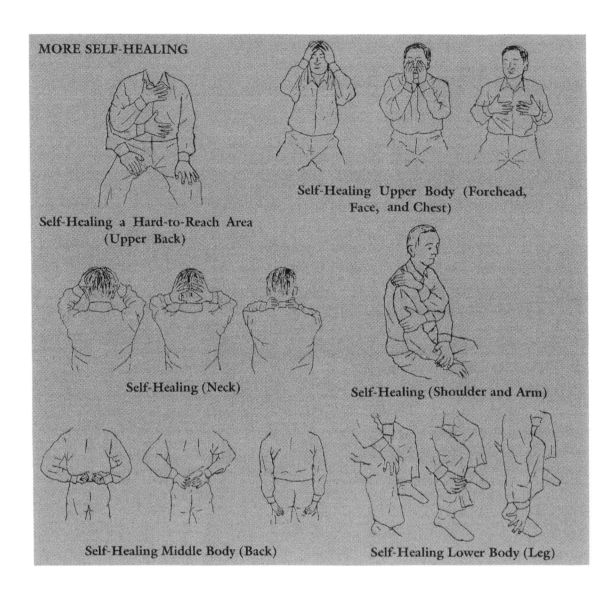

Self-Healing a Hard-to-Reach Area (Upper Back)

Self-Healing Upper Body (Forehead, Face, and Chest)

Self-Healing (Neck)

Self-Healing (Shoulder and Arm)

Self-Healing Middle Body (Back)

Self-Healing Lower Body (Leg)

## Self-Healing after Workouts

After seeing how four members of the Stanford Crew recovered from injuries and aches after learning one-with-nature touch for self-healing, the coach asked me to teach the whole team stress-reducing techniques to "cool down" after practice. First I taught the one-with-nature elements—relax, breathe, feel the earth, and do nothing extra. Then I taught them how to apply one-with-nature touch.

**Upper Body** To reduce stress in the forehead, face, and chest, place your palms on top of the head. Slowly lower your arms, bringing your palms down along the front of the body, from the face to the neck, the chest, and finally to the feet. While exhaling, feel the inner breath between the palms and body part being touched.

To reduce stress in the back of the head and neck, place your palms on top of your head again. Slowly lower your arms, bringing your palms down from the back of the head to the neck, the chest, and then to the floor. As you exhale, feel your inner breath between your palms and the body part being touched.

To reduce stress in the shoulder and arm, follow the same healing method.

**Middle Body**  To reduce stress in your back, make two fists and touch your back with the top of your fists in a circular motion several times. Then place your palms on your back and move them down toward your legs.

**Lower Body**  To reduce stress on one leg, begin by placing your hand on your knee and apply the same healing method.

This same self-healing method may be used to prevent injury caused by repeated motion, such as carpal tunnel syndrome, common among computer users. It can also reduce stress after strenuous workouts, or indeed after a hectic day at the office. It works for a wide range of discomforts like simple headaches, ulcers, menstrual cramps, tennis elbow, frozen shoulders, sprained wrists and ankles, and back injuries. The frequency with which you need to apply one-with-nature touch to achieve full healing will depend on the severity of the injury. This method is practical for healing injuries since it is easy to learn, has no side effects, and you do it yourself for free. But do not use it on open wounds, infections, or inflammations.

## Self and Nature

Nature heals us from both inside and outside. These diagrams might help you understand the relationship of the self to nature in natural healing.

The first diagram illustrates what you see when you look outward at nature, a very tiny self amid a vast natural world. The second diagram shows how you see nature when you look inward; the nature inside yourself seems much smaller than the grand me or self surrounding it. But if you look both inward and outward at the same time, you will be able to see nature and yourself as a whole. So, combining the first two diagrams into a third diagram, we have a tai chi, yin-and-yang symbol that illustrates this wholeness.

When you are one with nature, you realize that nature is part of you and that you, too, are part of nature. I observed during self-healing lessons that as I felt better, my students did also. I usually stop the lesson when I feel better. When we are in the one-with-nature state, everyone is the same since nature does not distinguish between you and me. So, what works for me will also work for you. We all have the ability to heal ourselves by

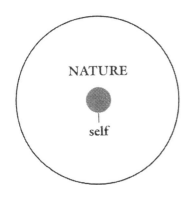   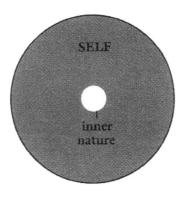   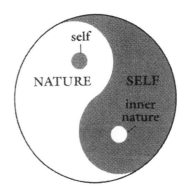

1  **Looking Outward at Nature**    2  **Looking Inward**    3  **The Yin and Yang of Tai Chi**

becoming one with nature.

Each time I see someone healed by becoming one with nature, I am amazed and thankful. Since nature is kind, being one with nature can perhaps make us kinder. As humanity becomes kinder, the world will be a more harmonious place to live in.

## Self-Healing and You

You can experience nature's kindness with self-healing. The next time you have an ache or injury, try this self-healing technique to feel better.

If you feel better, that means that the pain you felt was stress-related, which means that you were feeling unnecessary pain. By repeating this self-healing method you can reduce all unnecessary pain. If at the end of the self-healing session you still feel pain, what you're probably feeling is necessary pain. This is nature's signal that something is wrong and the area of pain demands your at-tention. But since every ache may have an unnecessary component, removing this component will help you feel better immediately. Self-healing is perhaps the kindest thing you can do for yourself.

### Self-Healing Technique
1. Touch the painful spot with your palm gently in a circular motion to make a thought–ch'i connection. Feel this spot with your palm and feel your palm moving on this spot, too, for a few minutes.
2. Cover the area with your palm lightly while you relax, breathe, feel the earth (floor), and do nothing extra for a minute or more.
3. Move your palm toward the floor down along your body, arm, or leg. Feel the touch between your palm and body while you exhale through your mouth gently.
4. Check to see if the painful spot feels better.

# CHAPTER SEVEN

# Personal Wellness and Cell Wellness

In these chapters we've presented ways to achieve inner happiness, self-control, self-realization, and self-healing. Over 5,000 of our tai chi students have benefited from the one-with-nature method. But what goes on inside the body and the mind that makes this work? When we unblock ch'i to enable its movement through the body, what happens physically? At the cellular level, what changes take place as you make yourself one with nature by relaxing, breathing, feeling the earth, and doing nothing extra? When your mind is with nature's mind, what enables each cell and organ and system to rid itself of stress?

Using the scientific method, we can develop or improve a theory or hypothesis and design experiments to test our theory. But even when repeatable experiments seem to prove a given theory, results can be equivocal or erroneous. If we approach the same problem in a different way with a different set of experiments, the original results may appear invalid.

Consider force and gravity. The one-with-nature element *feel the earth* can be restated "feel the earth's gravitational force in the body." This force was once measured in newtons, and scientists in the 18th and early 19th centuries believed, under Sir Isaac Newton's tutelage, that an object would gain more and more speed as more and more force was applied to it. But some 19th and 20th century scientists, like Albert Einstein, set about to disprove Newton's theory. Einstein's theory of relativity predicted that an object would gain more and more energy, rather than more speed, if more and more force was applied to it. And no object can travel faster than the speed of light.

The Stanford electron accelerator demonstrates the validity of Einstein's theory. An object, like an electron, can gain energy indefinitely as its speed increases toward the speed of light. Today many particle accelerators produce high-energy particle beams. Scientists use these beams to perform so-called high-energy physics experiments. In one such experiment, two particle beams collide. And through studies of this collision, we can develop new theories about the nature of forces which bind atomic nuclei together and eventually understand the elemental particles that compose the physical universe.

## Physical–Philosophical Study of the Self

We can also use the scientific method to study what I call *physical philosophy*. I first considered the philosophy behind tai chi, which I incorporated into my teaching and practice of tai chi, as described in our book *Ride the Tiger to the Mountain*. After devising the one-with-nature theory, I tried to verify it with experiments. And then I synthesized the knowledge gained from these experiments and formulated a new theory of cell control that's based on the one-with-nature theory.

## Cell-Wellness Theory

All the cells in the body originated from the division of another cell. Cell division, or mitosis, forms two cells identical to the parent cell from which both originated. These two cells are identical because just before division, all information and material in the parent cell is replicated. Each new cell has the same components as its parent cell.

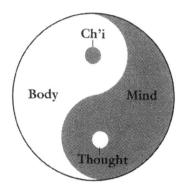

**The SELF or the CELL**

From conception, the human body has a set of cells and, as full adult beings, we are nothing more than an assembly of these cells. So, it seems logical to assume that if the four parts of the self—mind, body, thought, and ch'i—are present in the adult body, they're also present in each cell. That is, every cell may be said to contain a mind, body, thought, and ch'i of its own. The only real difference is that these four parts in each cell are seemingly less complex than they are in the self as a whole.

When the mind or body is under stress, the balance among the four parts of the self is disturbed and the flow of inner energy, or ch'i, is interrupted. When a cell is under stress, we may assume that the same thing occurs. And when a complex system of cells is out of balance—we could say that they're "unhappy"—stress-induced disorders such as tightness and pain are likely to result. Many disorders, like arthritis, allergies, and cancer, may be seen as caused by malfunctioning cells.

Cells in the nervous system, immune system, and cardiovascular system all appear to be specialized. We could say they all appear to have "minds of their own." Some cells communicate with each other to carry out specific tasks. G-proteins, for instance, act as go-betweens that translate messages into action inside cells. And it has been found that glia cells in the brain and spinal cord appear to nourish, protect, and listen to neu-

rons, and even talk back. These discoveries seem to support the hypothesis that each cell is in some way a microcosm of the self.

Within the self there is a natural connection between thought and ch'i. Since your cells are all part of yourself, the same connection must exist between every cell in the body and the self as a whole. In other words, your thoughts can influence the ch'i in each cell, and your ch'i can affect the thought of each cell.

If you are one with nature, then through the thought–ch'i connection each individual cell in your body could achieve the same state. We have already discussed self-healing, inner happiness, and self-control. Now we can talk about cell healing, cell happiness, and cell control. When a cell, just as when the self, is one with nature, it naturally achieves cell healing, cell happiness, and cell control.

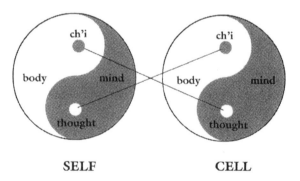

**SELF**         **CELL**

## New Cell-Wellness Experiments

With this theory, I understood how I was able to fully recover from allergies and asthma and how tai chi students had been able to recover from stress-related disorders. How does healing work at a cellular level, and what can cause a cell to be out of control? Stress inside the cell is one of the main causes, since that's when it becomes out of touch with nature. By using the inner breath, we can get rid of stress at the cellular level. When the cell is stress-free, it will be able to regain healing, happiness, and control. Perhaps it may even become more "intelligent."

To become one-with-nature we need to first learn the one-with-nature theory and basic methods, then practice them, and finally, apply them to wellness. These same steps seem necessary at the cellular level. Self-healing experiments described in an earlier chapter have involved mostly pain caused by stress. Pain, however, is difficult to measure. So, I began to look for new self-healing experiments that could produce quantifiable results, such as reduction of swelling and stiffness. Swelling and stiffness can be reduced almost immediately by using one-with-nature touch, with hands touching or *not* touching the body.

## Cell-Wellness Experiments with Touching
One-with-nature touch was used to reduce swelling for three tai chi students, one with a hand injured from falling, a second with an injured wrist, and a third with a swollen finger joint. For all three injuries, students were able to reduce swelling substantially within minutes. The first reduced swelling in the hand by about 60% within 7 minutes, the second in the wrist by 100% within 5 minutes, and the third in the finger joint by 50% within 5 minutes.

## Cell Wellness Experiments without Touching
This experiment allowed me to observe how fast tai chi students could reduce swelling and tightness in the nose, when this was caused by a cold or allergy.

### Reducing Swelling without Touching
- Sit comfortably.
- Relax, breathe, feel the earth (floor), and do nothing extra.
- Bring palm(s) near the forehead.
- Slowly move palm(s) down the face.
- When the palm(s) reach the nose, exhale through the mouth and feel the inner breath.
- Continue to move palm(s) down in front of the neck.
- Follow this warm feeling down the body.

This method can open air passages immediately. It can even stop a runny nose if it is applied before inflammation or a more serious condition occurs. Although this is not a cure for the common cold or for hay fever, it's probably the next best thing. It works because the cells are able to regain wellness without making physical contact with the body. It appears to verify the notion that we can control the cells through the natural connection between thought and ch'i.

Elayne, a tai chi student, had a terrible case of hay fever.

"When I walked into class, my nose had been stuffy and my eyes itching and red for two weeks. These signs reminded me of the serious hay fever I had suffered all through childhood and adolescence when I spent many uncomfortable days and nights with inflamed eyes and nose and had great difficulty breathing through my nose.

"Dr. Lee had me sit down and showed me how to pass my hand over my face and then down my body, by exhaling, keeping my wrist soft, feet on the ground, and body relaxed. After doing this several times using one hand, then the other, then both hands, my breathing eased and improved by about 65%. I then took the tai chi class. After 50 minutes, my breathing improved another 15% and my eyes were no longer red or itchy.

"During the next few days, whenever my nose began to feel stuffy, I practiced what Dr. Lee taught me. . . . A few moments of quiet practice would clear everything almost completely. This method sure beats antihistamines."

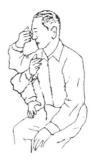

**Self-Healing without Touching**

## Cell-Healing and Cell Happiness

Today many alternative healing methods are available to treat different kinds of disorders. Many researchers have observed that relaxation is one of the most common prescriptions for healing stress-induced disorders, like depression, anxiety, digestive problems, high blood pressure, headaches, sprains or strains, insomnia, and arthritis.

Relaxation plays an important role in the healing process, and it seems to help prevent many stress-induced disorders in the first place. To achieve relaxation at the cellular level, we need to understand the connection between thought and ch'i. By practicing the one-with-nature elements—relax, breathe, feel the earth, and do nothing extra—we can enhance the thought–ch'i connection between our cells and ourselves. But remember, relaxation is only one of the one-with-nature elements. When combined, all four elements create a very powerful healing method indeed.

Using alternative healing methods, some people have reportedly recovered from cancer, undergoing total remission. Although these alternative methods are varied, they all seem to share a common factor, nature. Each alternative makes use of the natural connection of the self with nature to help us heal ourselves. Evidence of these various alternative healing methods offer us hope that we can heal ourselves or prevent development of diseases like cancer by becoming one with nature.

To what extent can we heal ourselves by becoming one with nature? Perhaps we need to experiment more. But it is clear that becoming one with nature is the fastest and easiest way to achieve healing and happiness. When you are in the one-with-nature state, whatever methods you use will work better and faster.

As you become one with nature, you can achieve not only cell healing but cell happiness as well. Think of the Chinese sage who in old age had the face of a happy child. To be happy like a child, every cell must be happy, like the cells of a child. As we achieve cell happiness, we can grow older without feeling old.

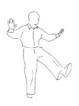

# CHAPTER EIGHT

# The Tao, Science, Philosophy, and Spirituality

East believes in nature and West believes in God. As for me, I believe in both God and nature. I am a part of nature; I also have a part of God in me. Inside me is both nature and God. I understand what people say about God, and I know what others write about nature—because I can be one with nature and with God. Being one with nature has helped me be one with God. It has removed pain from my body and saved me from the pain in my mind.

Like many of you, I've often wondered about the existence of a being greater than ourselves, the entity we know as God. From my wellness studies I've seen results that appeared miraculous. Students with serious ailments managed to heal themselves and seemed to awaken from disturbing pain to experience new heights. Each time I witnessed amazing results, I pondered the causes and concluded that the miracle came from something great inside the self. This existence found in the depths of the mind we might call the inner god.

The concept of the inner god should not be confused with the brain, which is simply a mechanism through which we express ourselves. We have tended to associate knowledge with the brain itself, since from birth the brain continually accumulates information. So, we conclude that the brain itself is responsible for this increase in knowledge. But the brain is really a tool that functions as a messenger between the mind and the physical world. The connections between mind and body and between thought and ch'i are similar to those formed between what we could call

your inner nature and inner god. These connections are so strong that I consider each bonded pair as two ways of looking at the same thing, or a duality.

This duality can easily be depicted by the yin-and-yang symbol. Although the two sides of the symbol share a common shape, they appear the opposite of each other. Yet together they form a whole and do not make sense on their own. With their unity they gain special significance. Yin and yang are two ways of looking at a whole, like the top and underside of your hand. Philosophers have pondered the duality of God and nature within and around us. And scientists have considered the duality of particles and waves as an expression of the duality of God and nature.

## Scientific Knowledge

The big bang theory helps explain how the universe was formed. And the theory of quantum mechanics, which involves the duality of particles and waves, helps support this theory. In Stephen Hawking's book *A Brief History of Time,* he wrote:

"The theory of quantum mechanics is based on an entirely new type of mathematics that no longer describes the real world in terms of particles and waves; it is only the observations of the world that may be described in those terms. There is thus a duality between waves and particles in quantum mechanics: for some purposes it is helpful to think of particles as waves and for other purposes it is better to think of waves as particles."

The most often cited examples of this duality of waves and particles are in experiments in optics, studies of light. In some experiments light behaves as particles, like tiny marbles, and in others, light acts like waves, much like those you see in oceans. Hawking says: "Up to now, most scientists have been too occupied with the development of new theories that describe what the universe is to ask the question why. On the other hand, the people whose business it is to ask why, the philosophers, have not been able to keep up with the advance of scientific theories. . . . If we find the answer to that, it would be the ultimate triumph of human reason—for then we would know the mind of God."

Scientists try to discover *how* the universe was created by a big bang. But philosophers ask *who* was responsible for the big bang. The scientist in me answers that it was nature that created itself. But if this is true, then how does God fit into the picture?

## Philosophical Knowledge

When reflecting on the duality of waves and particles, it occurred to me that God and nature are also a duality. Lao Tze describes the duality of tao that is central to Eastern philosophy: "Tao is the way, but it is not an ordinary way." Consider going to the store. The path is the road you take and the store is your destination. Considered in the ordinary way, the path and destination are different. But tao is not an ordinary way; it is both path and destination.

In this book, we have been concerned with reaching the destination we call one with nature. To achieve this state, we've involved ourselves in the process of being one with nature, or, if you prefer, becoming one with nature. But how can we be one with nature while being at the same time on our way to that destination?

Lao Tze, as I understand him, was talking about being one with our inner nature, the part of nature that's always within our bodies. If God is everywhere, then some part of God, like nature,

must also exist inside of you and me, in the mind just as nature resides in the body. The yin-and-yang symbol may be used to depict this duality of the inner God and inner nature.

## Inner Self

You can use thought to be with your inner god and ch'i to be with your inner nature. Remember that inner happiness is part of your thought and inner breath is part of your ch'i. We can also express this duality with the yin-and-yang symbol. Through meditation and the self-realization you may realize that inner god, inner nature, inner breath, and inner happiness are just four parts of the inner self.

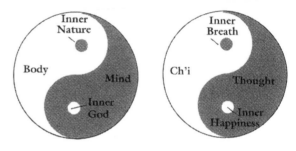

**INNER SELF**

## Tao and the Connection between Self and Inner Self

From the practice of the one-with-nature elements, you can use your mind, body, ch'i, and thought to achieve self-healing, inner happiness, self-control, and self-realization through relaxation, breathing, feeling the earth, and doing nothing extra. The process of looking inward and discovering what's there is known as tao.

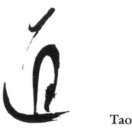

Tao

50

You can achieve the tao by being one with nature. When your mind is with the inner mind (the inner God), your body is with your inner body (nature), your ch'i is with your inner breath, and your thought is with your inner happiness. Through the process of looking inward you can realize the duality of the self and the inner self.

This is the inner path and destination for achieving what could be described as self-enlightenment. When you understand the tao, you will realize that there is no distinction between path and destination, mind and body, thought and ch'i, you and me, or even God and nature.

With knowledge of your inner self, you will be able to follow Buddha's advice: "Take the self as a lamp; take the self as a refuge. Betake yourselves to no external refuge. Hold fast as a refuge to the truth. Look not for refuge to anyone besides yourselves. Work out your own salvation with diligence."

## One with Nature for Humanity

It seems that everyone is under stress and indeed many are in distress. But how can we save ourselves and make the world a better place?

The world is, of course, a complex system, something like a person magnified many millions of times. The number of cells in a human being is comparable to the number of people in the world, counting in the billions. Since both the human body and the world community are composed of individual elements, they have, one might suppose, the same degree of complexity. Could the world community be out of touch with nature, just like an individual person in distress?

To create a better world, the human community must find a way to be one with nature just as individuals must. The world community needs to find a way to achieve global healing, global happiness, global control, and global realization. Because of the natural thought–ch'i connection between people, we can interact by using thought and ch'i.

We need to help each other become one with nature. And if all of humanity could become one with nature, we will help relieve and avoid much pain and suffering. Much can be achieved with nature's help.

It may seem naïve to think that techniques so simple as those discussed in this book combined

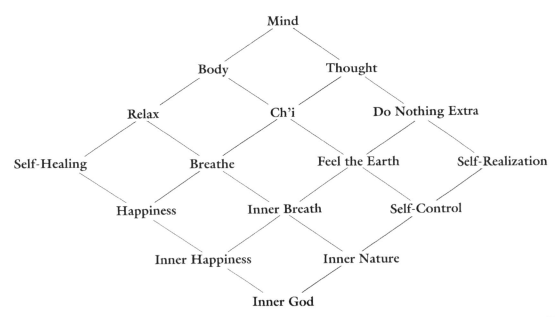

with our own natural abilities can achieve events of global merit. But we are just one thought away from making the world a better place to live in. As Buddha said: "We are what we think. All that we are arises with our thought. With our thoughts we make the world. Speak or act with a pure mind and happiness will follow you as your shadow, unshakable."

## Self-Enlightenment

Everyone knows there is only one nature. Not everybody thinks there is a God. Supposing God is related to nature, there must be also one God. God does not ask why, nor does God ask why not. To God, there is not any difference between why and why not. There is only being. Nature does not say what is, nor does nature say what is not. In nature, there is no distinction between what is and what is not. There is only existence. Since both God and nature are inside me, I can understand my own existence and being by looking inward. Tao is being one with nature, and spirituality is being one with God. For me, the attainment of both tao and spirituality is enlightenment.

# CHAPTER NINE

# Beginner's Guide to Tai Chi Practice

To help you learn one-with-nature tai chi, we present sixty-four individual lessons, traditionally called forms. This sequence of forms is based on Yang-style tai chi, developed by Yang Pan-Hou (1837–1892). Each form is a lesson complete in itself with written instructions and illustrations for one or more movements. Most forms, like Wind Blows Lotus Leaves, have just one movement or part, but others, like Work the Shuttle in the Clouds, have as many as four.

Freeze-action photos demonstrate each movement in four stages (*a* to *d*). Note the arrow below the photo for the direction of movement. Also observe the two drawings for the form's "start" and "end" positions. The *a* position in the photo and instructions refers to the start position and the *d* position to the end position for that particular movement. For forms with more than one movement, the final movement's *d* position is the end position for that form.

Practice each form in a continuous motion. Since each form continues into the next, the start position for the form is the end position of the preceding form. By learning the forms in the order presented here, your tai chi exercises will be smooth, uninterrupted, and like slow dance. With practice, you will be able to perform all sixty-four one-with-nature tai chi forms in about ten to twelve minutes. Daily practice of these movements, enhanced by one-with-nature elements (relax, breathe, feel the earth, and do nothing extra) will strengthen the natural connections between mind, body, ch'i, and thought.

Some forms, like Single Whip and Wave Hands Like Clouds, are repeated in the sequence of sixty-four forms. Although the start positions—*a*—vary according to the preceding form, the movement—most of *b* and all of *c* and *d*—will be the same. So, once you learn these forms, you will be able to practice them with confidence in graceful sequence.

Grand Tai Chi is a form independent of the sequence of sixty-four, but you should end every practice session of tai chi with this form. You can also practice Grand Tai Chi by itself to help you relax and feel energized at any time of day. Grand Tai Chi offers essential benefits, such as calming, healing, and strenghtening, which will help you become one with nature.

Whenever you practice one-with-nature tai chi, keep these things in mind.

**Warm-Up** It's always a good idea to do gentle rotation exercises for your joints and gentle stretching exercises for your muscles and tendons before you begin tai chi.

**Body Orientation** Imagine yourself in the center of a square or a square room. The end position of each form should always be the same, defined by one of these directions: front, rear, left, right, right front corner, right rear corner, left front corner, and left rear corner. See pp. 56–59 for the body's orientation, given in parentheses, under the drawing of the end position of each of the sixty-four forms.

**Relaxation** Relaxation is crucial in the practice of tai chi. Relax every part of your body, inside and out.

**Breathing**   Breathe smoothly and regularly, allowing the tai chi movements to regulate your breathing pattern. Pay attention to exhaling and do not hold your breath. Let your whole body be involved in the breathing process. Learn to feel your breath through all parts of the body.

**Attention (Feeling)**   Be aware of what you are doing—your movement, breathing, relaxation, and distribution of weight. Monitor the entire process to be sure that you are feeling the earth and doing nothing extra.

**Intention (Thinking)**   Be mindful of each movement, and when you have learned a movement, calm your mind and allow your mind to lead you through it. Think before and as you move. Allow your mind to direct your movement.

**Posture**   Keep your torso upright but relaxed and look straight ahead. Don't lean to one side, bend excessively forward or back, or look down. It is also important not to overextend your limbs or clench your hands into tight fists. Tai chi is a natural art that requires no excessive force and no harsh intentions. Keep in mind that this exercise is slow and calm. You do not need to forcefully push, punch, or kick. Leave that to the active combat of other martial arts.

**Symmetry**   The right leg should remain on the right side of the body and the left leg on the left. As you step forward or backwards, don't let your feet cross the centerline of your body.

**Shifting Weight**   In tai chi your weight is often on one leg at a time. To shift weight from one leg to another, use your intention. However, you should feel balanced by staying centered as you shift weight from a solid, weight-bearing leg to a hollow, nonweight-bearing leg.

At other times when your weight is fairly even on both legs, this is called "sitting in the middle."

**Pace**   Move at the same slow-and-relaxed pace through every movement. Tai chi has been traditionally described as the slow unwinding of a silky filament of a silkworm's cocoon.

**Practice**   Each day practice all the movements you have learned up to that date. Practice them in sequence several times. Do not practice immediately after a meal. Also, it's best to wear loose clothing and flat shoes.

**Checklist**   You should feel comfortable while performing all the movements. Make sure that with each movement your shoulders are down and your knees remain slightly bent, never locked. Your hands and wrists should always be loose and relaxed with palms open and fingers slightly apart.

- If your neck is uncomfortable, check to see if it is relaxed.
- If your shoulders are uncomfortable, check to make sure they are loose.
- If your arms are uncomfortable, check to see if they are overextended, out too far or up too high.
- If your legs are uncomfortable, check to see if they are bent too much or they are too close or too far from each other.

Carefully read the instructions for each movement of each form and observe the start and end positions in the two drawings. Also look at the four images in the photo that accompanies each movement for the *a*, start position, and *d*, end position. The two intermediate positions, *b* and *c*, are transitional. As you become familiar with each movement, you will not need to stop or pause at these transitional positions. And, as the circles around the drawings advise, relax, breathe, feel the earth, and do nothing extra. Direct your attention to your body's movements and your mind's intention to performing them.

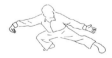

# The 64 Forms of One-with-Nature Tai Chi

*Illustrations on pp. 56–59 show end positions with body orientation in parentheses.*

1. Pay Respect to Buddha (Humankind)
2. Grasp the Bird's Tail
3. Single Whip
4. White Crane Spreads Its Wings
5. Brush Knees and Twist Step
6. Deflect, Parry, and Punch
7. Apparent Close Up
8. Carry the Tiger to the Mountain
9. Under Elbow Blow
10. Step Back to Repulse the Monkey
11. Slanted Palms Flying
12. Raise Right and Left Hands
13. Step Up with Flying Arm
14. Fan across Shoulder
15. Green Dragon Rises from Water
16. Single Whip
17. Wave Hands Like Clouds
18. Single Whip
19. High Pat on Horse
20. Right and Left Split Kick
21. Turn Around and Heel Kick
22. Wind Blows Lotus Leaves
23. Block Up and Punch Down
24. Turn Around and Double Kick
25. Step, Deflect, Parry, and Punch
26. Step and Pull Back
27. Face Front and Kick
28. Turn Around and Heel Kick
29. Step, Deflect, Parry, and Punch
30. Apparent Close Up
31. Embrace the Tiger
32. Pull and Push with Body
33. Diagonal Single Whip
34. Parting the Wild Horse's Mane
35. Diagonal Single Whip
36. Work the Shuttle in the Clouds
37. Turn and Grasp the Bird's Tail
38. Single Whip
39. Wave Hands Like Clouds
40. Single Whip Down
41. Golden Rooster Stands on One Leg
42. Step Back to Repulse the Monkey
43. Slanted Palms Flying
44. Raise Right and Left Hands
45. Step Up with Flying Arm
46. Fan across Shoulder
47. Push and Box Ears
48. Firing Cannon into the Sky
49. Single Whip
50. Wave Hands Like Clouds
51. Single Whip
52. High Pat on Horse
53. Wave Cross at Water Lily
54. Fist Pounding Down
55. Turn and Grasp the Bird's Tail
56. Single Whip
57. Wave Hands Like Clouds
58. Single Whip Down
59. Step to Reach Seven Stars
60. Retreat to Ride the Tiger
61. Slant Body to Rock the Moon
62. Wave Lotus Foot
63. Pulling Bow to Shoot an Arrow
64. Right and Left Grasp the Bird's Tail

Grand Tai Chi

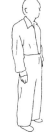

**Grand Tai Chi (*front*)**

# End Positions of the 64 Forms with Body Orientation

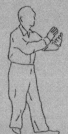 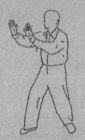 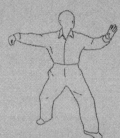 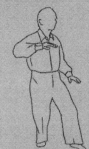

1. Pay Respect to Buddha (*front*)

2. Grasp the Bird's Tail (*right front corner*)

3. Single Whip (*front*)

4. White Crane Spreads Its Wings (*left*)

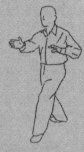 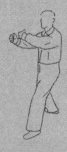 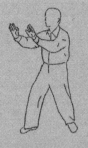 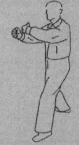

5. Brush Knees and Twist Step (*left*)

6. Deflect, Parry, and Punch (*left*)

7. Apparent Close Up (*left*)

8. Carry the Tiger to the Mountain (*right*)

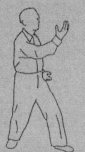 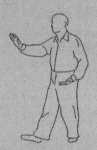 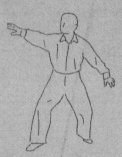 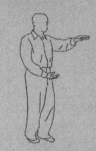

9. Under Elbow Blow (*right*)

10. Step Back to Repulse the Monkey (*right*)

11. Slanted Palms Flying (*front*)

12. Raise Right and Left Hands (*rear*)

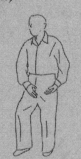 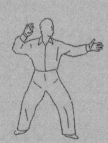 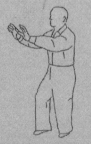 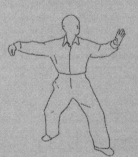

13. Step Up with Flying Arm (*rear*)

14. Fan across Shoulder (*rear*)

15. Green Dragon Rises from Water (*left rear corner*)

16. Single Whip (*rear*)

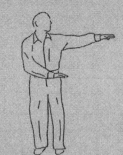 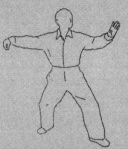 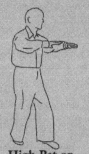 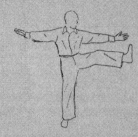

**17. Wave Hands Like Clouds** (*rear*)  **18. Single Whip** (*rear*)  **19. High Pat on Horse** (*right*)  **20. Right and Left Split Kicks** (*right*)

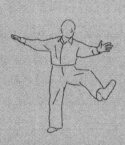 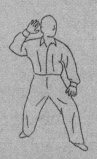 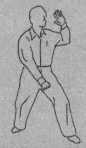 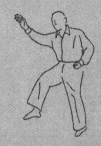

**21. Turn Around and Heel Kick** (*left front corner*)  **22. Wind Blows Lotus Leaves** (*left rear corner*)  **23. Block Up and Punch Down** (*left rear corner*)  **24. Turn Around and Double Kick** (*right front corner*)

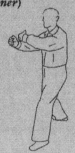 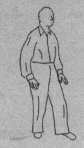 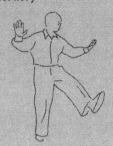 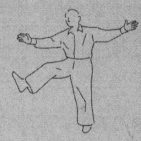

**25. Step, Deflect, Parry, and Punch** (*right front corner*)  **26. Step and Pull Back** (*right front corner*)  **27. Face Front and Kick** (*right front corner*)  **28. Turn Around and Heel Kick** (*left front corner*)

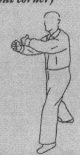 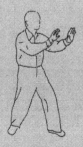 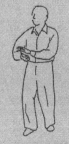 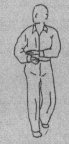

**29. Step, Deflect, Parry, and Punch** (*right front corner*)  **30. Apparent Close Up** (*right front corner*)  **31. Embrace the Tiger** (*left rear corner*)  **32. Pull and Push with Body** (*left rear corner*)

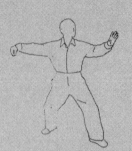

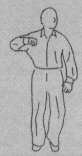

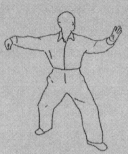

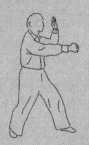

**33. Diagonal Single Whip** (*left rear corner*)

**34. Parting the Wild Horse's Mane** (*left rear corner*)

**35. Diagonal Single Whip** (*left rear corner*)

**36. Work the Shuttle in the Clouds** (*right rear corner*)

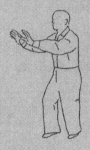

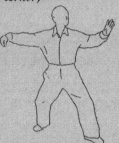

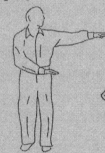

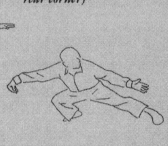

**37. Turn and Grasp the Bird's Tail** (*left rear corner*)

**38. Single Whip** (*rear*)

**39. Wave Hands Like Clouds** (*rear*)

**40. Single Whip Down** (*rear*)

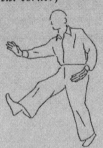

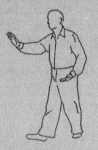

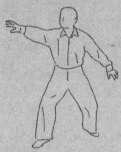

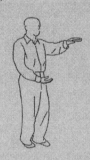

**41. Golden Rooster Stands on One Leg** (*right*)

**42. Step Back to Repulse the Monkey** (*right*)

**43. Slanted Palms Flying** (*front*)

**44. Raise Right and Left Hands** (*rear*)

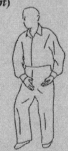

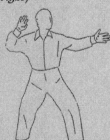

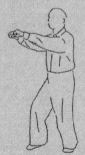

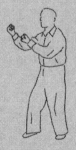

**45. Step Up with Flying Arm** (*rear*)

**46. Fan across Shoulder** (*rear*)

**47. Push and Box Ears** (*right*)

**48. Firing Cannon into the Sky** (*right*)

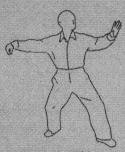

**49. Single Whip**
(*front*)

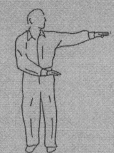

**50. Wave Hands Like Clouds** (*front*)

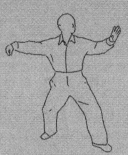

**51. Single Whip**
(*front*)

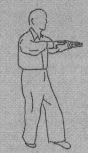

**52. High Pat on Horse** (*left*)

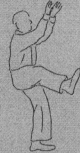

**53. Wave Cross at Water Lily** (*left*)

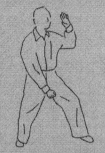

**54. Fist Pounding Down** (*left*)

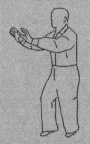

**55. Turn and Grasp the Bird's Tail** (*left rear corner*)

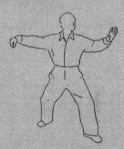

**56. Single Whip** (*rear*)

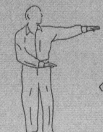

**57. Wave Hands Like Clouds** (*rear*)

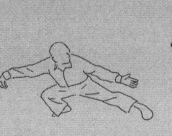

**58. Single Whip Down** (*rear*)

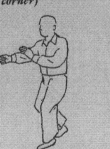

**59. Step to Reach Seven Stars** (*right*)

**60. Retreat to Ride the Tiger** (*right*)

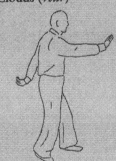

**61. Slant Body to Rock the Moon** (*rear*)

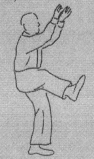

**62. Wave Lotus Foot** (*front*)

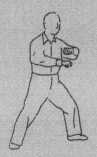

**63. Pulling Bow to Shoot Arrow** (*front*)

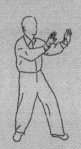

**64. Right and Left Grasp the Bird's Tail** (*left front corner*)

# One-with-Nature Tai Chi
# the 64 Forms

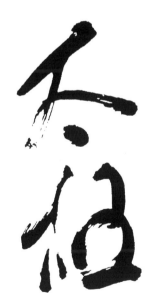

# 1. Pay Respect to Buddha (Human- kind)

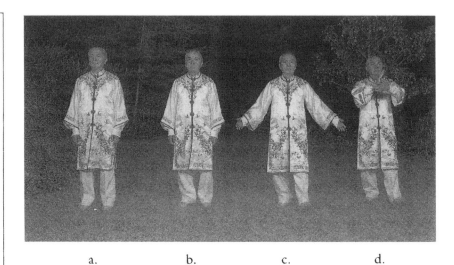

a.       b.       c.       d.

**Starting Position (Get Ready)** Stand with feet parallel, knees slightly bent, and arms along sides with palms open facing body.

*Intention and Attention:* Relax, breathe, feel the earth, and do nothing extra. *All 64 forms involve these one-with-nature elements.*

## Movement

**a.** Start from the "get ready" position, relax, breathe, feel the earth, and do nothing extra.

**b.** Turn your right foot out 45° and shift your weight to the right leg.

**c.** Bring left foot forward with heel down. Open palms and bring hands out to waist height.

**d.** Raise arms up in front of your chest with your left palm facing the body, and your right palm facing left, right fingers pointing up, and elbows the same height from the ground.

**End Position** The right foot turns out 45° with knee bent, and the left foot rests on heel in front of hip. Arms form a circle.

*Intention:* Block with left arm, monitor block with right arm; and feel the body's weight on right leg.

*Attention:* Relax, breathe, feel the earth, and do nothing extra. Attend to how you feel inside.

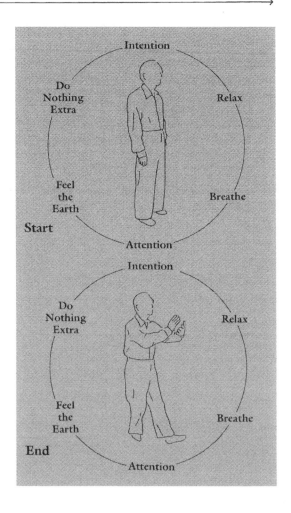

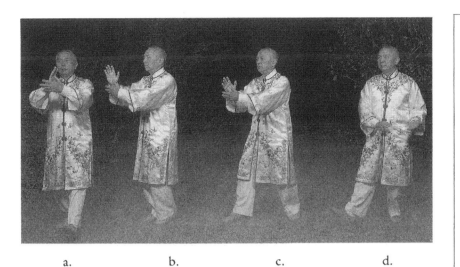

a.  b.  c.  d.

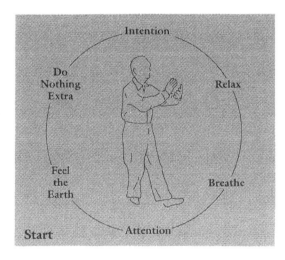

Intention

Do Nothing Extra

Relax

Feel the Earth

Breathe

**Start**  Attention

## Movement (First Part)

**a.** Starting position is the end position from Pay Respect to Buddha (Humankind).

**b.** Turn body right 45°. Bring left foot near body. Turn the right palm down and the left palm up.

**c.** Step back with left foot.

**d.** Shift weight to left leg and lift up toes of right foot. Bring both hands down to left side.

*continued*

# Grasp the Bird's Tail

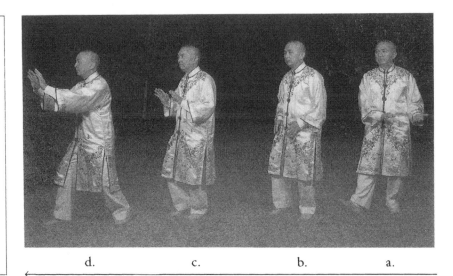

| d. | c. | b. | a. |

## Movement (Second Part)

**a.** Start from *d* above.

**b.** Bring right foot near body and move hands in front.

**c.** Bring arms up to chest level with palms facing forward.

**d.** Step with right foot and push hands forward. Weight should be even on both legs.

**End Position**   Right foot points forward and left foot turns out 60° with knees evenly bent.

*Intention:* Push with both arms and feel the body weight even on both legs.

*Attention:* Relax, breathe, feel the earth, and do nothing extra. Attend to how you feel inside.

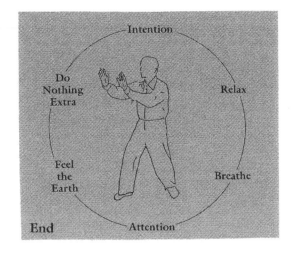

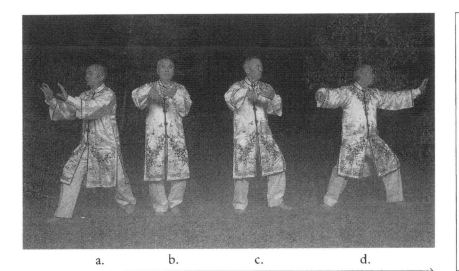

a.    b.    c.    d.

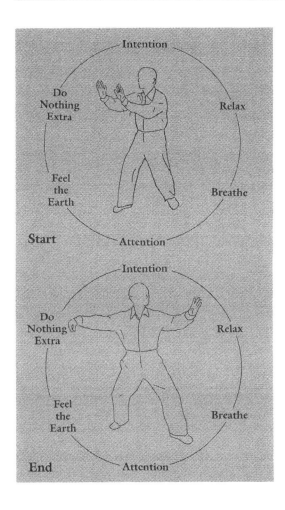

## Movement

**a.** Starting position is the end position from Grasp the Bird's Tail.

**b.** Turn body and right foot left 45° and bring left foot near the body. Shift weight to the right leg. Bring both hands in front near the body. The right hand forms a beak and the left palm turns toward the body.

**c.** Turn head toward the left, and turn left foot and step left with the left foot. Move hands out in a circle.

**d.** Bend both knees, lowering the body slightly. Push the left hand toward the left and extend the right arm toward the right.

**End Position**   Right foot points forward and left foot points left. The head turns left and the left hand pushes to the side. The right hand forms a beak; knees are bent evenly.

*Intention:* Push left arm, grasp right arm, and feel body weight even on both legs.

*Attention:* Relax, breathe, feel the earth, and do nothing extra. Attend to how you feel inside.

# 4. White Crane Spreads Its Wings

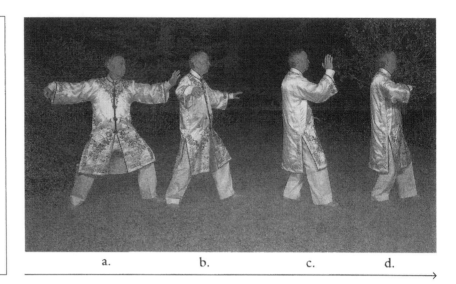

a.  b.  c.  d.

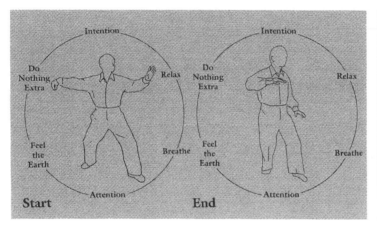

Start  End

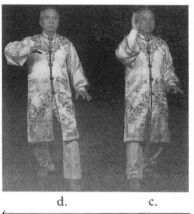

d.  c.

**Side View**

## Movement

**a.** Starting position is the end position from Single Whip.

**b.** Turn the body left 90° and both feet left 45°. Shift your weight to the left leg with knees bent.

**c.** Step forward with right foot and bring the right hand forward with palm facing left. Lower the left hand to the waist with palm down.

**d.** Move the right foot near the body, and step with the right foot toward right with toes pointing out 45°. Shift weight to the right leg, and bring left foot in front of the hip. Push the right elbow to the side and extend left elbow back slightly (also see side view).

**End Position**   Right foot turns out 45° and left foot points forward. Left elbow aims backward with hand along side, palm down. Right elbow aims at the side with hand in front. Knees are bent.

*Intention:* Push with both arms and feel body weight on the right leg.

*Attention:* Relax, breathe, feel the earth, and do nothing extra. Attend to how you feel inside.

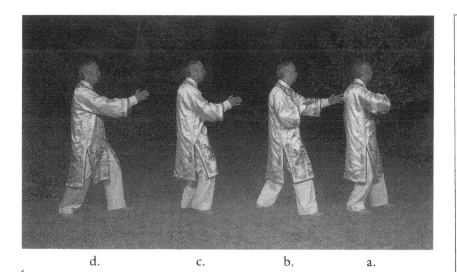

d.          c.          b.          a.

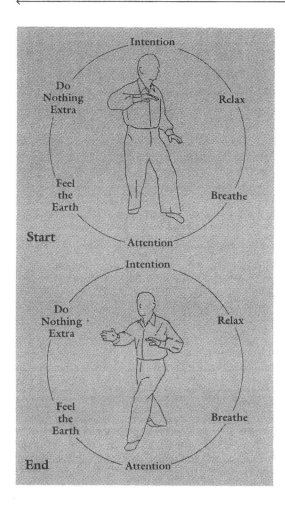

**Start**

Intention · Relax · Breathe · Attention · Feel the Earth · Do Nothing Extra

**End**

Intention · Relax · Breathe · Attention · Feel the Earth · Do Nothing Extra

## Movement

**a.** Starting position is the end position from White Crane Spreads Its Wings.

**b.** Step back with the left foot. Push palms to the right below shoulder height, left hand in front of right hand along your side. Weight is even on both legs with knees slightly bent.

**c.** Shift weight to the left leg and move the right foot near the body. Bring both hands to the left side.

**d.** Step back with the right foot. Push palms to the left below shoulder height, with the right hand in front of the left hand along your side. Weight is even on both legs and knees are slightly bent.

**End Position** Feet turn out 30° with knees bent evenly. Hands are along the left side with the right palm in front of left palm and fingers pointing forward.

*Intention:* Pull with left arm, push with right arm, and feel body weight even on both legs.

*Attention:* Relax, breathe, feel the earth, and do nothing extra. Attend to how you feel inside.

67

# 6.
# Deflect, Parry, and Punch

❦

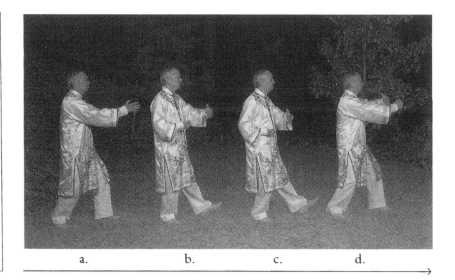

a.    b.    c.    d.

## Movement

**a.** Starting position is the end position from Brush Knees and Twist Step.

**b.** Shift weight to right leg and lift up left toes. Make a fist with right hand and bring it toward right side near the body, knuckles down. Sweep the left hand toward body in an arc, with the palm facing the body.

**c.** Bring the left hand near body and begin to raise right fist.

**d.** Step forward with the left foot and turn right foot out 60° with both knees evenly bent. Move left forearm slightly forward and punch right arm under left forearm (not touching) to complete the movement with body weight even on both legs.

**End Position** Turn right foot out 60° and point left foot forward with knees bent evenly. Right hand makes a fist, and left hand faces the body (above right forearm).

*Intention:* Deflect with left arm, punch with right arm, and feel body weight even on legs.

*Attention:* Relax, breathe, feel the earth, and do nothing extra. Attend to how you feel inside.

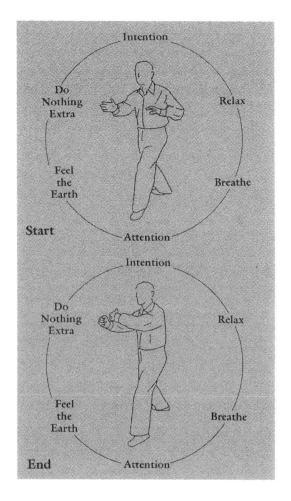

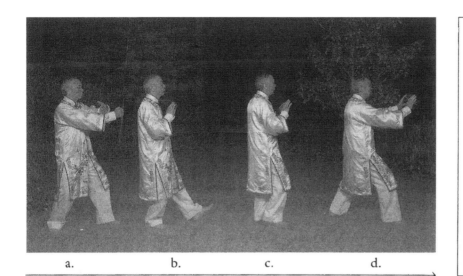

a.    b.    c.    d.

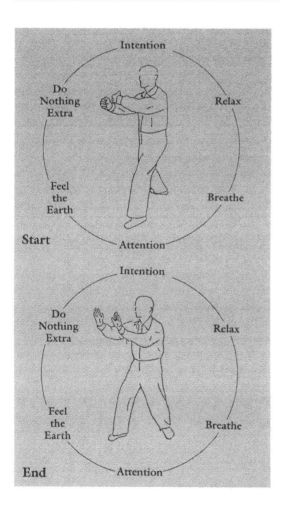

Start

End

## Movement

**a.** Starting position is end position from Deflect, Parry, and Punch.

**b.** Shift weight to the right leg and lift up left toes. Pull both hands toward the chest with palms facing forward.

**c.** Shift weight to left leg and bring right foot forward near the left foot.

**d.** Step forward with right foot, bend knees, and push hands forward. Weight is even on both legs.

**End Position** Left foot turns out 60° and right foot points forward with knees bent evenly. Both arms extend almost fully with palms facing forward.

*Intention:* Push with both arms and feel body weight even on both legs.

*Attention:* Relax, breathe, feel the earth, and do nothing extra. Attend to how you feel inside.

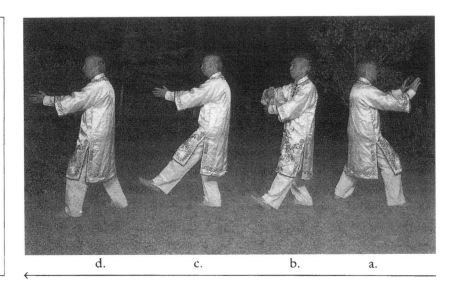

## 8. Carry the Tiger to the Mountain

🌿

| d. | c. | b. | a. |

## Movement (First Part)

**a.** Starting position is the end position from Apparent Close Up.

**b.** Turn body left 180° and right foot out 45°. Shift weight to right leg, move left foot in front of hip, and rest foot on heel. Make right fist and turn left palm toward body. Bring hands in front to form circle with right fist above left palm.

**c.** Lift left foot up slightly and bring both hands forward with left hand in front of right hand and fingers pointing forward.

**d.** Step down with the left foot. Bring both hands toward right side and move arms from right to left with hands making the lower half of a circle, clockwise.

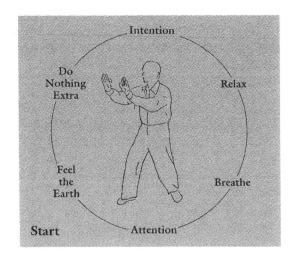

70

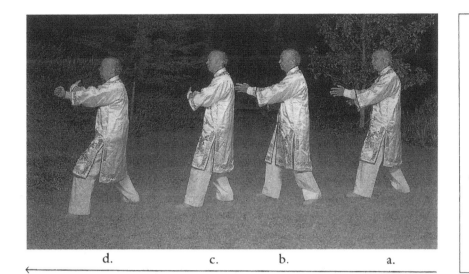

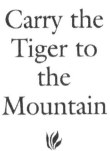

# Carry the Tiger to the Mountain

d.      c.      b.      a.

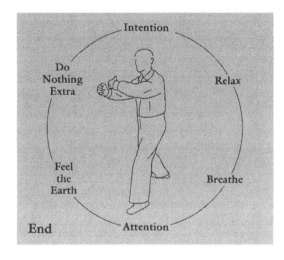

## Movement (Second Part)

**a.** Start from *d* above.

**b.** Step forward with right foot. Bring both hands from left toward right side making upper half of a circle, clockwise.

**c.** Make a fist with right hand and bring it toward right side near waist with knuckles down. Sweep left hand toward the body in an arc.

**d.** Step forward with left foot with both knees bent. Shift body weight evenly on legs. Move left arm forward and punch right arm under left forearm with fist upright.

**End Position** Right foot turns out 60° and the left foot points forward with knees bent evenly. Right arm extends forward under the left wrist (not touching). Left palm faces the body and the right hand makes a fist.

*Intention:* Deflect left arm, punch right arm, and feel body weight even on both legs.

*Attention:* Relax, breathe, feel the earth, and do nothing extra. Attend to how you feel inside.

71

# 9. Under Elbow Blow

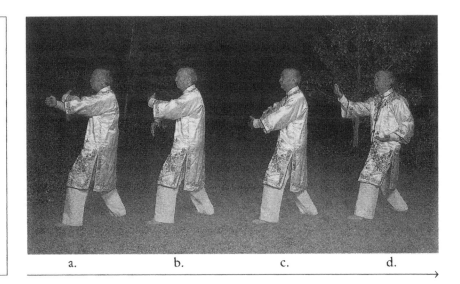

a.       b.       c.       d.

## Movement

**a.** Starting position is the end position from Carry the Tiger to the Mountain.

**b.** Open right fist and bring right hand under left hand with the right palm facing the body.

**c.** Begin lowering the left hand to the left side, palm up.

**d.** Move the right hand up and forward with elbow bent, and bring left hand to left waist. Palms are up.

**End Position**  Right foot turns out 60° and left foot points forward with knees bent evenly. Right hand faces body and left hand is alongside, palm up.

*Intention:* Strike with right arm, pull with left arm, and feel body weight even on both legs.

*Attention:* Relax, breathe, feel the earth, and do nothing extra. Attend to how you feel inside.

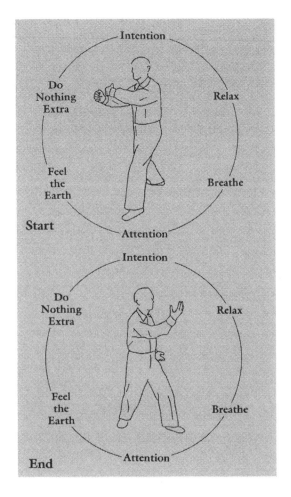

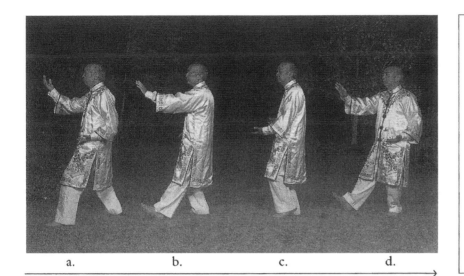

a.  b.  c.  d.

## 10. Step Back to Repulse the Monkey

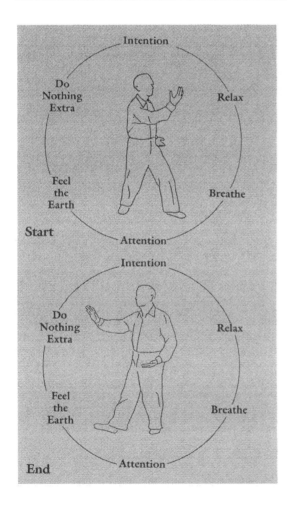

**Intention**

Do Nothing Extra

Relax

Feel the Earth

Breathe

**Start**

Attention

**Intention**

Do Nothing Extra

Relax

Feel the Earth

Breathe

**End**

Attention

## Movement

**a.** Starting position is the end position from Under Elbow Blow.

**b.** Shift weight to right leg and lift left toes up. Turn right palm down and pull it back to the waist. Bring the left hand up and push it forward. Arm and leg positions are the same as *d* with right and left interchanged.

**c.** Bring the left foot near the body. Begin to bring the right hand up. Turn the left palm up and bring it down to the waist.

**d.** Step back with your left foot out 45°. Shift weight to the left leg and lift your right toes up. Push the right hand forward, palm out, and pull the left hand to the waist, palm up.

**End Position**   Left foot turns out 45° and right foot rests on heel. Right hand extends forward with palm out and left hand is along waist with palm up.

*Intention:* Push with right arm, pull with left arm, and feel the body's weight on the left leg.

*Attention:* Relax, breathe, feel the earth, and do nothing extra. Attend to how you feel inside.

73

# 11.
# Slanted
# Palms
# Flying

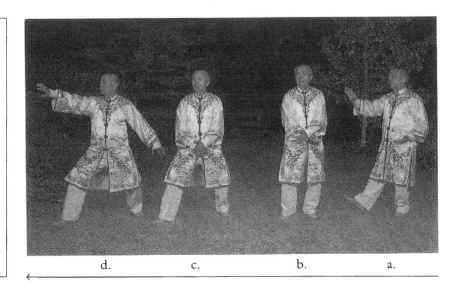

d.　　　c.　　　b.　　　a.

## Movement

**a.** Starting position is the end position from Step Back to Repulse the Monkey.

**b.** Turn left foot and body 45°. Bring right foot near left foot with toes pointing out 45°, and bring both hands in front of the body with the left wrist above the right wrist. Shift weight to the left leg.

**c.** Step 45° toward the right. Shift weight to both legs with bent knees.

**d.** Sweep arms outward, raising the right arm to shoulder height and the left arm to hip level with palms facing back.

**End Position**   Both feet turn out 45° and knees are bent. Extend both arms along sides, slanted, with palms facing back.

*Intention:* Sweep with right arm, deflect with left arm, and feel the body's weight on both legs.

*Attention:* Relax, breathe, feel the earth, and do nothing extra. Attend to how you feel inside.

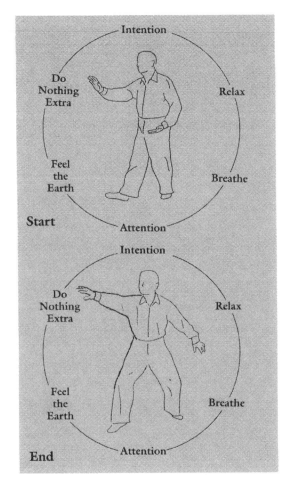

74

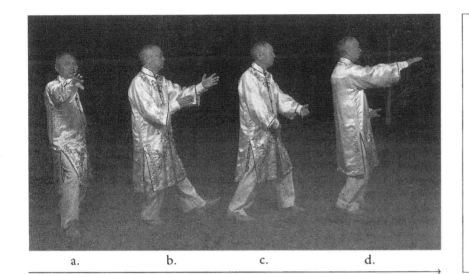

a.      b.      c.      d.

## 12. Raise Right and Left Hands

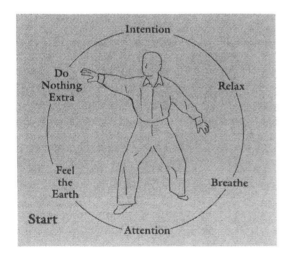

## Movement (First Part)

**a.** Starting position is the end position from Slanted Palms Flying.

**b.** Shift weight to the right leg, and bring left foot in front of hip. Rest on heel. Move both arms forward, palms in.

**c.** Step down with left foot forward. Lower the left hand with palm up and lower the right hand with palm down.

**d.** Shift the body's weight to the left leg. Bring the right foot near the left foot along the side with the heel up. Raise the right arm and lower the left hand in front of the body. Arm and leg positions are the same as shown in *d* in the second part of this movement, with right and left interchanged.

*continued*

# Raise Right and Left Hands

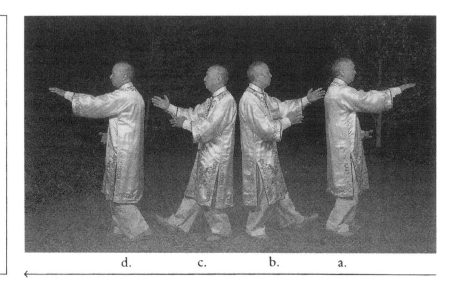

d.    c.    b.    a.

## Movement (Second Part)

**a.** Start from the end position of the first part of this movement.

**b.** Step back with right foot. Lift up the left toes and shift weight to the right leg. Lower the right hand and move the left arm forward along the sides in front of the body, palms in.

**c.** Turn body toward the right 180° and turn on the heel of your left foot 135°. Step down with the left foot. Shift weight to the left leg, and move the right foot slightly to the side, in front of the hip and rest on the heel. Lower the left hand and move the right arm forward.

**d.** Step down on the right foot and shift the body's weight to the right leg. Bring the left foot near the right foot along the side with the heel up. Raise the left arm and lower the right hand in front of the body.

**End Position**  Left foot is behind the right foot along the side, with the left heel up. The

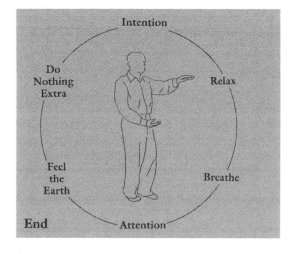

left hand points forward at shoulder height, with palm down, and the right hand is in front of the body, palm up.

*Intention:* Push with left arm, block with right arm, and feel the body's weight on the right leg.

*Attention:* Relax, breathe, feel the earth, and do nothing extra. Attend to how you feel inside.

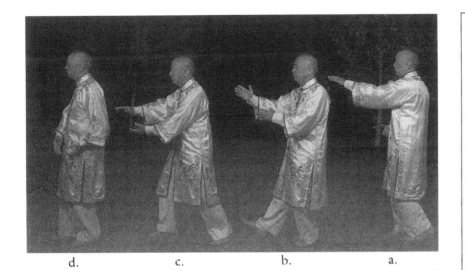

d.　　　　c.　　　　b.　　　　a.

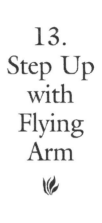

# 13.
# Step Up with Flying Arm

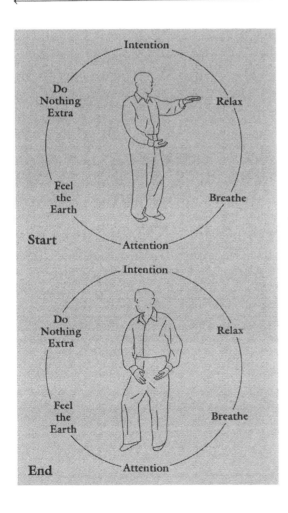

Start

End

## Movement

**a.** Starting position is the end position from Raise Right and Left Hands.

**b.** Step back with left foot, with the foot turned out 45°. Shift the body's weight to the left leg and lift up right toes. Lower the left hand to chest height and move the right arm forward with palms in and fingers pointing forward.

**c.** Step forward with right foot, and reach forward with both hands, right above left, right palm down and left palm up.

**d.** Shift weight to the left leg. Bring the right foot back near the left foot with the right heel up. Pull both hands near the body, waist level along the left side with palms facing each other.

**End Position**   The left foot is 45° out and the right heel up. The right arm crosses the body at 45° and palms face each other.

*Intention:* Deflect down with the right arm, pull with left arm, and feel the body's weight on the left leg.

*Attention:* Relax, breathe, feel the earth, and do nothing extra. Attend to how you feel inside.

## 14. Fan across Shoulder

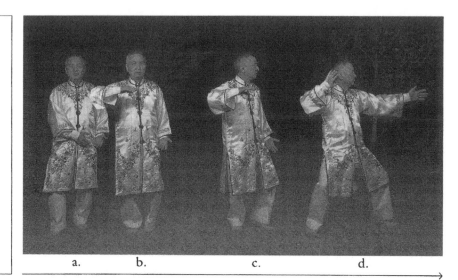

a.   b.   c.   d.

## Movement

**a.** Starting position is the end position from Step Up with Flying Arm.

**b.** Step forward with right foot. Bring left foot near the right foot, and lift up the left heel and shift weight to the right leg. Raise the right forearm to shoulder height, palm down.

**c.** Turn the head to look left. Turn the left foot and left hand toward the left.

**d.** Step with left foot toward the left. Raise the left hand to shoulder height with fingers pointing left, and bring your right hand up to temple level with palm out.

**End Position**   Left foot turns 90° out and right foot points forward. Left hand points left at shoulder level, and right hand covers the head at temple height.

*Intention:* Push out with the left arm, pull back with the right arm, and feel the body's weight on both legs.

*Attention:* Relax, breathe, feel the earth, and do nothing extra. Attend to how you feel inside.

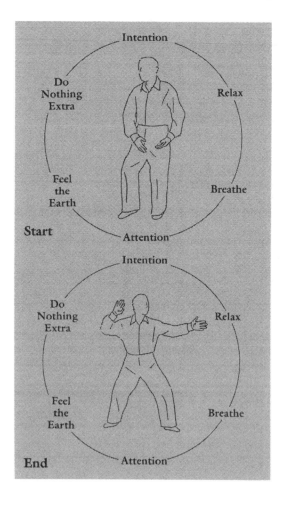

78

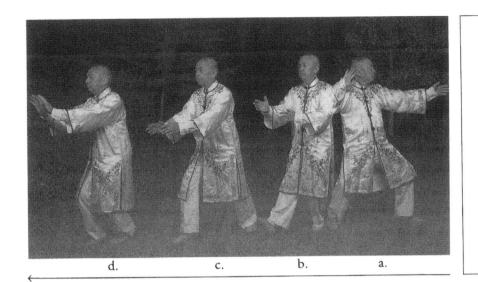

d.      c.      b.      a.

## 15. Green Dragon Rises from Water

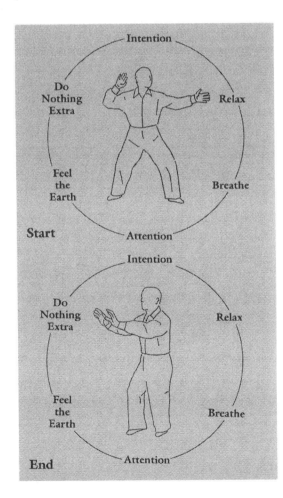

Intention

Do Nothing Extra      Relax

Feel the Earth      Breathe

**Start**      Attention

Intention

Do Nothing Extra      Relax

Feel the Earth      Breathe

**End**      Attention

## Movement

**a.** Starting position is the end position from Fan across Shoulder.

**b.** Turn the body and left foot 45° clockwise. Bring the right foot in front of hip and rest it on the heel. Raise both hands to chest height, with the right hand in front of the left and fingers pointing forward. Shift weight to the left foot.

**c.** Step down with the right foot, and bend knees. Reach forward with both hands, with palms facing each other.

**d.** Bring the right foot near the left foot, and bring both hands toward the body with fingers pointing forward. Shift weight to the left leg. Step forward with the right foot and follow with the left foot. Push both hands forward with the body weight on both legs.

**End Position**   Right foot is in front of the left foot. Knees are bent, and palms face forward.

*Intention:* Push forward with both arms and feel the body's weight on both legs.

*Attention:* Relax, breathe, feel the earth, and do nothing extra. Attend to how you feel inside.

# 16.
# Single Whip

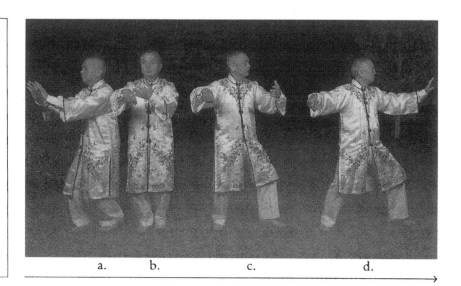

a.　　b.　　c.　　d.

## Movement

**a.** Starting position is the end position from Green Dragon Rises from Water.

**b.** Turn the body and left foot 45° toward the left. Shift weight to the right leg. Bring both hands in front of the body. The right hand forms a beak and the left palm turns toward the body.

**c.** Turn head toward the left, and turn left foot and step left with the left foot. Move hands out in a circle.

**d.** Bend both knees, lowering the body slightly. Push the left hand toward the left and extend the right arm toward the right.

**End Position** Right foot points forward and left foot points left. The head turns left and the left hand pushes to the side. The right hand forms a beak; knees are bent evenly.

*Intention:* Push left arm, grasp right arm, and feel body weight even on both legs.

*Attention:* Relax, breathe, feel the earth, and do nothing extra. Attend to how you feel inside.

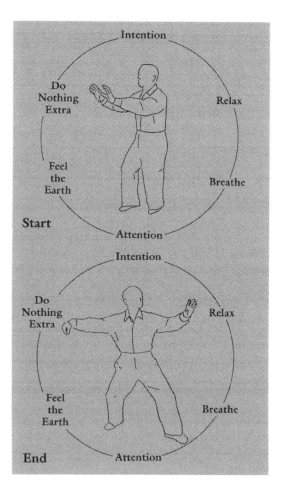

80

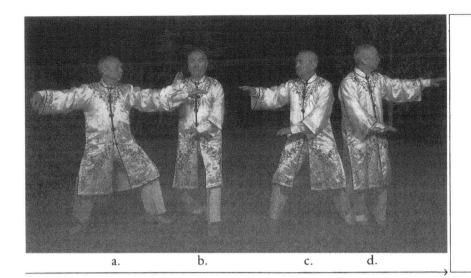

# 17. Wave Hands Like Clouds

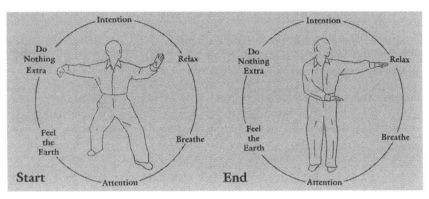

a.      b.      c.      d.

Start

End

## Movement

**a.** Starting position is the end position from Single Whip.

**b.** Turn right foot out 45° and shift weight to the right leg. Move the left foot in front, with heel up. Bring hands in front of the body with palms down. The right hand is at chest height and left hand hip-level.

**c.** Step toward left side with the left foot and turn the right foot parallel to the left foot. Turn the head to look right. Move the right hand toward the right side at shoulder height and the left hand in front of the right hip, palms down. Keep weight even on both legs and bend knees slightly.

**d.** Bring right foot near the left foot. Raise the left hand up and across to shoulder height. Move the right hand down to hip level with body weight even on both legs.

**End Position**   Head turns toward left. Feet are parallel and knees bent evenly. The left arm extends toward the left at shoulder height, palm down, and the right arm is in front of the body near the left hip, palm down.

*Intention:* Sweep with left arm, deflect with right arm, and feel the body's weight on both legs.

*Attention:* Relax, breathe, feel the earth, and do nothing extra. Attend to how you feel inside.

# 18. Single Whip

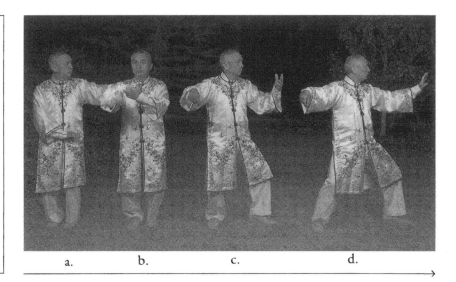

a.      b.      c.      d.

## Movement

**a.** Starting position is the end position from Wave Hands Like Clouds.

**b.** Turn the head to look forward and shift weight to the right leg. Bring both hands in front of the body. The right hand forms a beak and the left palm turns toward the body.

**c.** Turn head toward the left, and turn left foot and step left with the left foot. Move hands out in a circle.

**d.** Bend both knees, lowering the body slightly. Push the left hand toward the left and extend the right arm toward the right.

**End Position**    Right foot points forward and left foot points left. The head turns left and the left hand pushes to the side. The right hand forms a beak; knees are bent evenly.

*Intention:* Push left arm, grasp right arm, and feel body weight even on both legs.

*Attention:* Relax, breathe, feel the earth, and do nothing extra. Attend to how you feel inside.

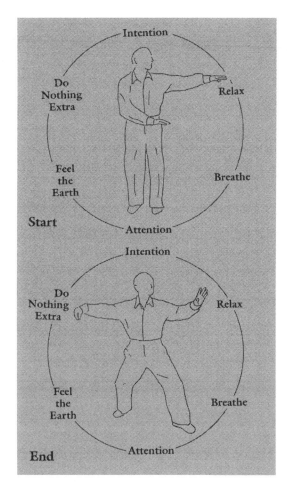

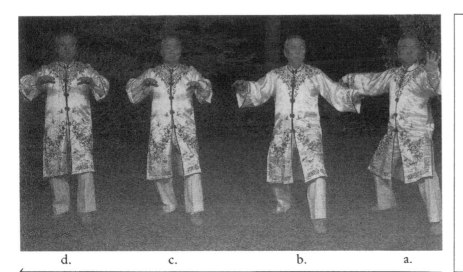

d.        c.        b.        a.

# 19. High Pat on Horse

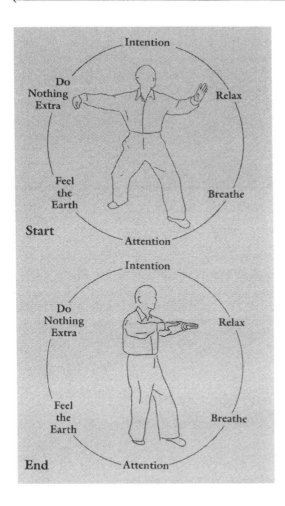

Start

End

## Movement

**a.** Starting position is the end position from Single Whip.

**b.** Turn the body and the right foot 45° toward the left.

**c.** Shift weight to the right leg and bring the left foot in front of the hip, with heel up. Move both hands in front of the chest, palms down.

**d.** Bend knees and complete the movement with the body's weight on the right leg.

**End Position** Right foot is out 45° and the left heel up; knees are bent. Hands are in front of the chest, arms in a circle and palms down.

*Intention:* Block with the left arm, hold with the right arm, and feel the body's weight on the right leg.

*Attention:* Relax, breathe, feel the earth, and do nothing extra. Attend to how you feel inside.

# 20. Right and Left Split Kick

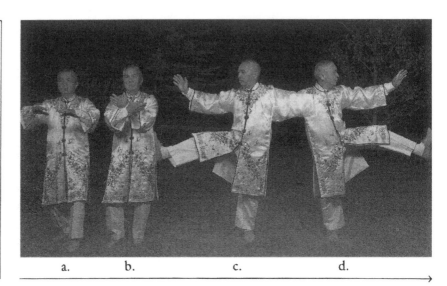

a.　　　b.　　　　c.　　　　d.

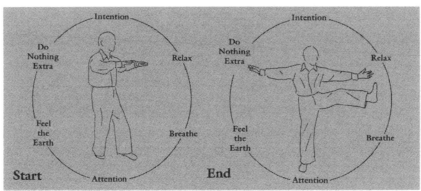

## Movement

**a.** Starting position is the end position from High Pat on Horse.

**b.** Step forward with the left foot, and bring the right foot near the left foot with the right heel up and right toes pointing out. Shift your weight to the left leg. Cross hands in front with palms facing the body, the right hand in front of the left hand.

**c.** Turn your head to look right. Turn palms toward the front and move arms up and out in a circle. Kick with your right foot upward along the right side. The leg position is the same as *d* with right and left interchanged.

**d.** Step down with right foot near the left foot.

Shift weight to the right leg with the left heel up and left toes pointing out. Cross hands in front with palms facing the body, left hand in front of right hand. Turn the head and look left. Turn palms toward the front and move arms up and out in a circle. Kick the left foot upward along the left side.

**End Position**　Head turns toward the left and the left foot kicks to the side, with right knee bent. Arms spread open and palms face forward.

*Intention:* Block with both arms, kick with left leg, and feel the body's weight on right leg.

*Attention:* Relax, breathe, feel the earth, and do nothing extra. Attend to how you feel inside.

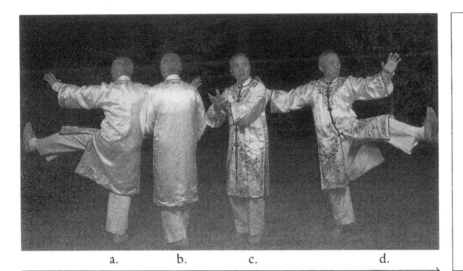

a.     b.     c.       d.

## 21. Turn Around and Heel Kick

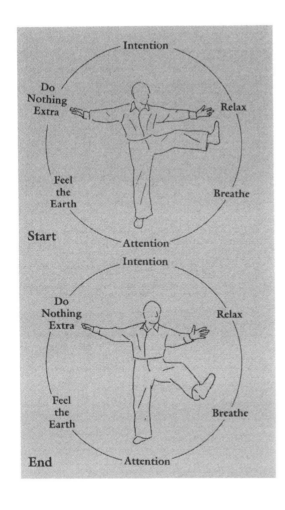

**Start**

**End**

## Movement

**a.** Starting position is the end position from Right and Left Split Kick.

**b.** Step down with the left foot behind the body and cross your hands in front, with palms facing the body.

**c.** Turn the body and the right foot 135° toward the left (a three-eighths turn counterclockwise). Shift the weight to the right leg and lift up the left heel.

**d.** Point left toes out. Turn both palms facing forward and move the arms up and out in a circle. Kick with left heel up and to the side.

**End Position**    Kick left foot to the side and push with the heel. The arms are open and the right knee bent.

*Intention:* Block with both arms, kick with the left leg, and feel the body's weight on the right leg.

*Attention:* Relax, breathe, feel the earth, and do nothing extra. Attend to how you feel inside.

## 22. Wind Blows Lotus Leaves

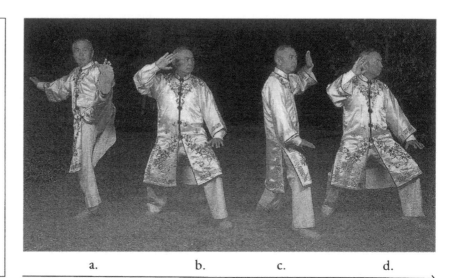

a.       b.       c.       d.

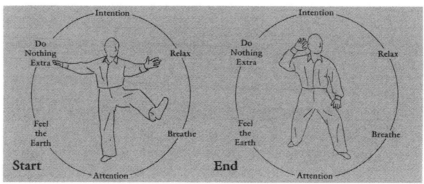

## Movement

**a.** Starting position is the end position from Turn Around and Heel Kick, facing the left back corner of the room.

**b.** Step forward with left foot, toes pointing forward and the weight on both legs. Bring the left hand down, with palm down, along the front of the body, and the right hand up toward the temple. Arms and legs are the same as in *d* below.

**c.** Turn the left foot 45° out and step forward with the right foot. Shift the weight onto both legs and bend both knees. Bring the left hand up to the temple, and move the right hand down along the front of the body above the right knee. Arms and legs are the same as in *d* below, with right and left interchanged.

**d.** Turn the right foot 45° out and step forward with the left foot. Move the left hand down, with palm down, in front of the body above the left knee, and move the right hand up toward the temple. Bend both knees. Complete this movement with the weight even on both legs.

**End Position**  Right foot turns out 60° and the left foot points forward, with knees bent evenly. Left hand is above knee, palm down, and right hand is near the temple, palm out.

*Intention:* Sweep down with the left arm, block up with the right arm, and feel the body's weight on both legs.

*Attention:* Relax, breathe, feel the earth, and do nothing extra. Attend to how you feel inside.

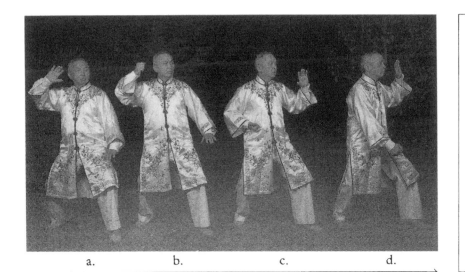

a.       b.       c.       d.

# 23.
# Block Up and Punch Down

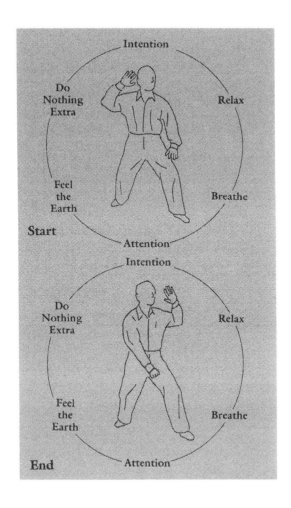

## Movement

**a.** Starting position is the end position from Wind Blows Lotus Leaves.

**b.** Make right fist and bring left hand up slightly.

**c.** Lower the right hand down toward left leg, and bring left hand toward temple.

**d.** Bend both knees evenly and punch with the right fist.

**End Position**   Right foot turns out 60° and left foot points forward, with knees bent evenly. Left hand is near temple, palm out, and the right arm extends downward on the right side of the body parallel to the left leg.

*Intention:* Block with the left arm, punch with the right arm, and feel the body's weight even on both legs.

*Attention:* Relax, breathe, feel the earth, and do nothing extra. Attend to how you feel inside.

## 24. Turn Around and Double Kick

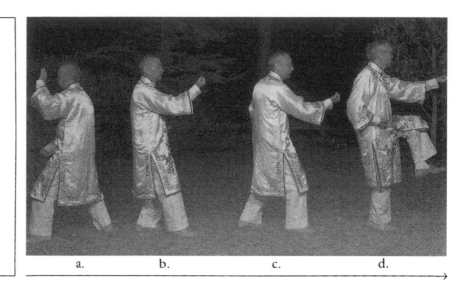

a.    b.    c.    d.

## Movement (First Part)

**a.** Starting position is the end position from Block Up and Punch Down.

**b.** Turn the body 180° and the left foot 135°, both clockwise. Make a left fist and shift the weight to the left foot, bringing the right foot in front of the hip, heel up. Bring right fist up and out in front of the body at shoulder height and the left fist near the waist.

**c.** Step forward with right foot, and shift the weight to the right leg.

**d.** Raise the left knee up with the foot parallel to the floor. Push the left arm forward, fist turned up, and bring the right fist to the waist.

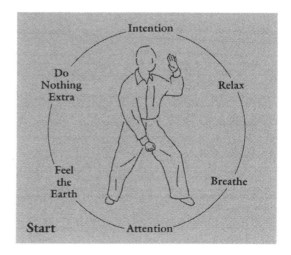

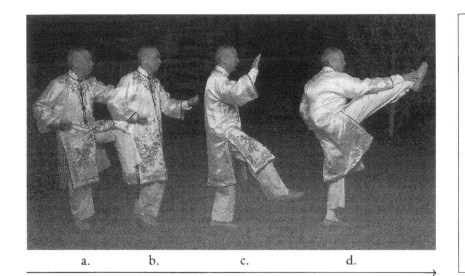

a.   b.   c.   d.

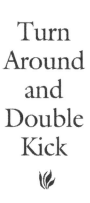

# Turn Around and Double Kick

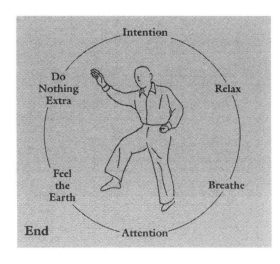

Intention

Do Nothing Extra

Relax

Feel the Earth

Breathe

End

Attention

## Movement (Second Part)

**a.** Start from position *d* above.

**b.** Step forward slightly with left foot and shift weight to the left leg.

**c.** Open the right fist and bring the right hand up and out with the palm facing forward. Bring the left fist to the waist, and bring the right foot upward ready to kick.

**d.** Complete the right foot's kick and slap the right palm toward the right leg.

**End Position**   Right foot kicks up and right hand strikes forward toward right leg. The left fist is along the side at waist-height.

*Intention:* Strike with right arm, pull with left arm, kick with right leg, and feel the weight on the left leg.

*Attention:* Relax, breathe, feel the earth, and do nothing extra. Attend to how you feel inside.

# 25.
# Step, Deflect, Parry, and Punch

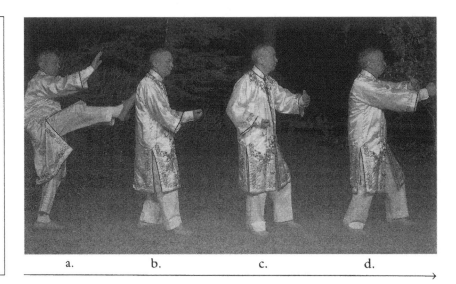

a.   b.   c.   d.

## Movement

**a.** Starting position is the end position from Turn Around and Double Kick.

**b.** Step down with right foot out 45°. Make a right fist and bring it toward the body with knuckles down. Sweep the left hand toward the body in an arc.

**c.** Move the left palm in front of body, the right fist near the chest along the side, and bring the left foot forward.

**d.** Complete step forward with left foot and turn the right foot out 60°. Bend both knees and shift the weight so that it's even on both legs. Move the left forearm forward slightly and punch with the right arm under the left forearm with arms not touching.

**End Position**   The right foot turns out 60° and the left foot points forward, with knees bent evenly. The right hand makes a fist, and the left hand faces the body above the right forearm.

*Intention:* Deflect with the left arm, punch with the right arm, and feel the body's weight even on both legs.

*Attention:* Relax, breathe, feel the earth, and do nothing extra. Attend to how you feel inside.

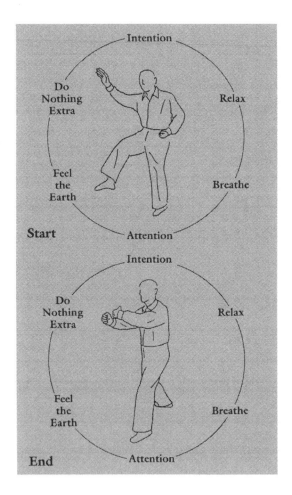

90

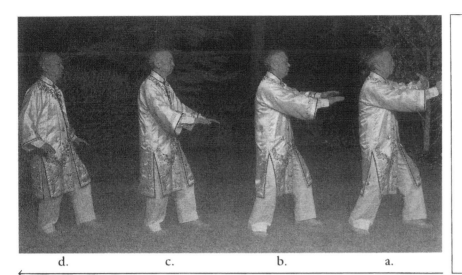

d.        c.        b.        a.

# 26. Step and Pull Back

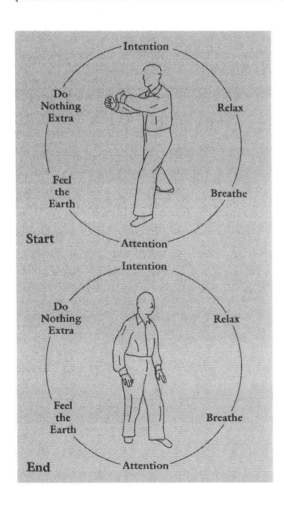

## Movement

**a.** Starting position is the end position from Step, Deflect, Parry, and Punch.

**b.** Open right fist.

**c.** Step backward with right foot and bring the left foot along, heel up, shifting weight to the right leg. Pull hands backwards.

**d.** Bring both hands to the side, palms down, to complete the movement.

**End Position**    Right foot turns out 45° and left foot points forward, heel up. Knees are bent; both palms face down along the sides.

*Intention:* Pull back with both arms and feel the body's weight on the right leg.

*Attention:* Relax, breathe, feel the earth, and do nothing extra. Attend to how you feel inside.

## 27. Face Front and Kick

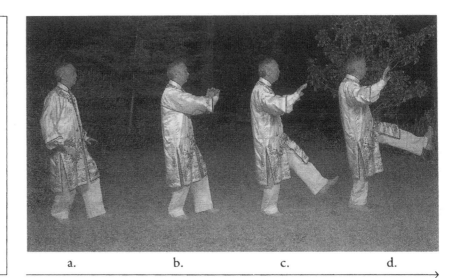

a.     b.     c.     d.

## Movement

**a.** Starting position is the end position from Step and Pull Back.

**b.** Bring arms up in front of body, palms down, and move the left foot toward the body slightly, heel up.

**c.** Cross the hands in front with palms facing forward, and kick left leg forward and up.

**d.** Sweep arms up and out to complete the movement.

**End Position**   Right foot turns out 45° and left foot kicks forward. Right knee is bent and both arms swing open with palms facing forward.

*Intention:* Block with both arms, kick with left leg, and feel the body's weight on the right leg.

*Attention:* Relax, breathe, feel the earth, and do nothing extra. Attend to how you feel inside.

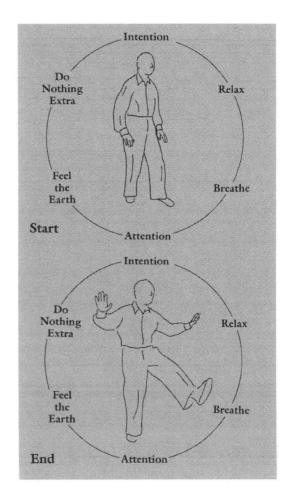

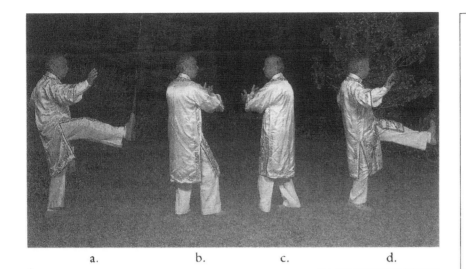

a.    b.    c.    d.

## 28. Turn Around and Heel Kick

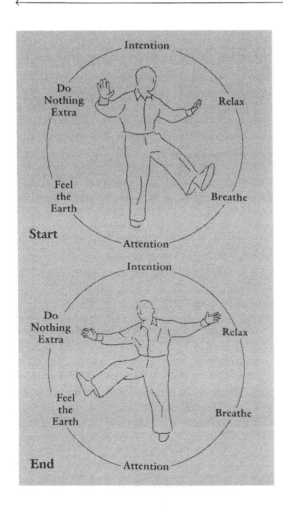

**Start**

**End**

## Movement

a. Starting position is the end position from Face Front and Kick.

b. Lower left foot and turn body and right foot clockwise 135° (three-eighths turn). Step down on the left foot in front of the right toes to form a "T". Cross both hands in front of the chest with palms facing in.

c. Turn the body and the right foot 135° toward the right (a three-eighths turn clockwise). Shift the weight to the left leg and lift up the right heel.

d. Point right toes out. Turn both palms facing forward and move the arms up and out in a circle. Kick with right heel up and to the side.

**End Position**   Kick right foot to the side and push with the heel. The arms are open and the left knee bent.

*Intention:* Block with both arms, kick with the right leg, and feel the body's weight on the left leg.

*Attention:* Relax, breathe, feel the earth, and do nothing extra. Attend to how you feel inside.

93

## 29. Step, Deflect, Parry, and Punch

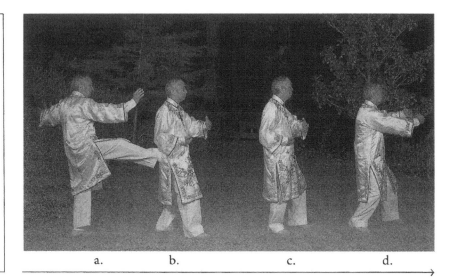

a.    b.    c.    d.

## Movement

**a.** Starting position is the end position from Turn Around and Heel Kick.

**b.** Turn body 45° toward the right and step forward with the right foot. Make a fist with right hand and bring it to the side near the body (with knuckles down). Sweep the left arm toward the body in an arc.

**c.** Move the left palm in front of body, the right fist near the chest along the side, and bring left foot forward.

**d.** Complete step forward with left foot and turn the right foot out 60°. Bend both knees and shift the weight so that it's even on both legs. Move the left forearm forward slightly and punch with the right arm under the left forearm with arms not touching.

**End Position** The right foot turns out 60° and the left foot points forward, with knees bent evenly. The right hand makes a fist, and the left hand faces the body above the right forearm.

*Intention:* Deflect with the left arm, punch with the right arm, and feel the body's weight even on both legs.

*Attention:* Relax, breathe, feel the earth, and do nothing extra. Attend to how you feel inside.

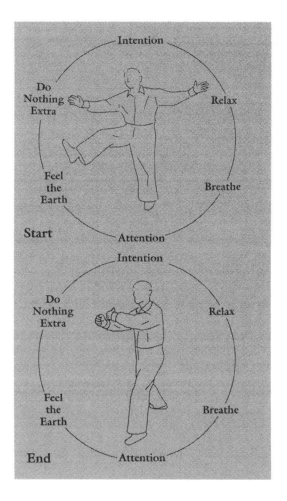

94

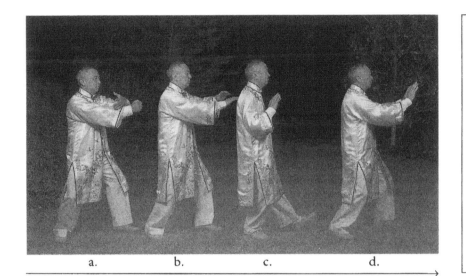

a.　　　b.　　　c.　　　d.

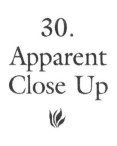

## 30. Apparent Close Up

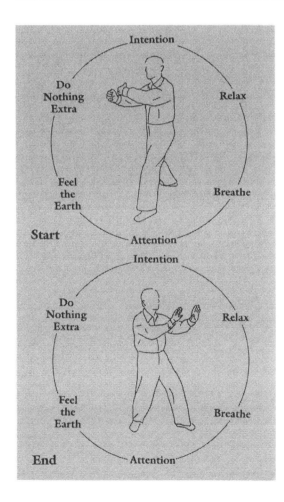

Start

End

## Movement

**a.** Starting position is the end position from Step, Deflect, Parry, and Punch.

**b.** Open the right fist and move hands toward the chest, palms out.

**c.** Shift weight to the right leg, and lift up the the left toes. Bring both hands up in front of the chest with palms facing forward.

**d.** Step down with the left foot and turn the right foot out 60°. Bend both knees evenly. Push both hands forward to complete this movement with the weight even on both legs.

**End Position**　Right foot turns out 60° and the left foot points forward; knees are evenly bent. Both arms extend almost fully and palms face forward.

*Intention:* Push with both arms and feel the body's weight on both legs.

*Attention:* Relax, breathe, feel the earth, and do nothing extra. Attend to how you feel inside.

95

## 31. Embrace the Tiger

🌿

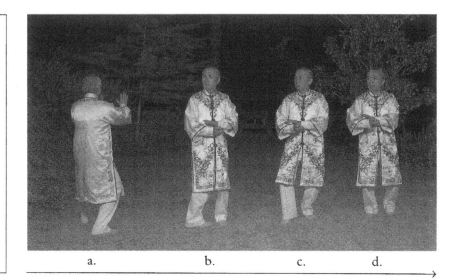

a.　　　b.　　　c.　　　d.

## Movement

**a.** Starting position is the end position from Apparent Close Up.

**b.** Shift weight to your right leg and turn the body right 90°. With your left foot, step in front of the right foot to form a "T". Knees are bent. Make a fist with your right hand, knuckles down, and place the left palm above the right wrist, not touching. Bring your hands near the body.

**c.** Shift weight to the left leg, lift up the right heel, and turn the body while turning the right foot 180° clockwise.

**d.** Step forward with the right foot, and bring the left foot near right foot with heel up. Shift weight onto both legs with knees slightly bent, and push both arms forward.

**End Position**   Left foot turns out 60° and the right foot points forward, with knees bent evenly.

*Intention:* Push with right forearm and left hand, and feel the body's weight on both legs.

*Attention:* Relax, breathe, feel the earth, and do nothing extra. Attend to how you feel inside.

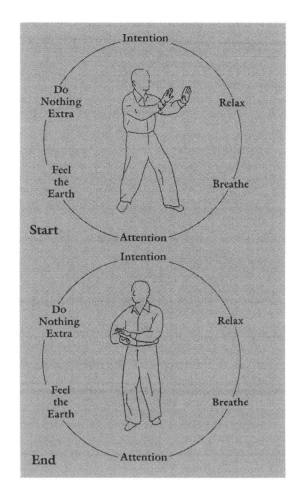

96

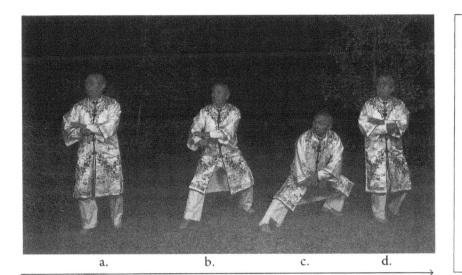

a.    b.    c.    d.

## 32. Pull and Push with Body

🔥

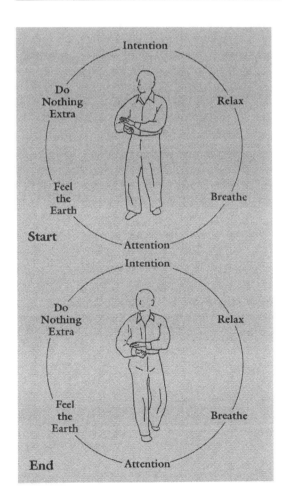

Intention

Do Nothing Extra

Relax

Feel the Earth

Breathe

**Start**

Attention

Intention

Do Nothing Extra

Relax

Feel the Earth

Breathe

**End**

Attention

## Movement

**a.** Starting position is the end position from Embrace the Tiger.

**b.** Step backwards with left foot, with toes pointing out 90°.

**c.** Lower body and turn the right foot 90°, parallel to the left foot. Rotate the right fist in toward the body and pull hands down as the body is lowered.

**d.** Raise the body up, and shift weight to the right leg with heel up. Rotate the right fist outward, and push arms forward.

**End Position**   Right foot aims forward and left heel is up. Make a fist with the right hand, knuckles down. Left hand is above right forearm, not touching.

*Intention:* Push with both arms and feel the body's weight on both legs.

*Attention:* Relax, breathe, feel the earth, and do nothing extra. Attend to how you feel inside.

## 33. Diagonal Single Whip

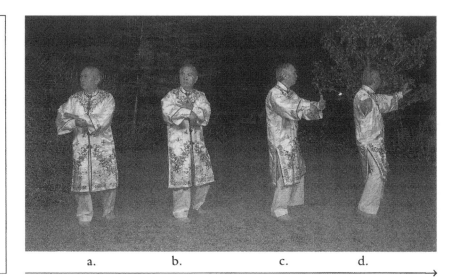

a.　　　b.　　　c.　　　d.

## Movement

**a.** Starting position is the end position from Pull and Push with Body.

**b.** Turn the body toward the left 45°. Bring left hand up in front of the body. Right fingers form a beak and left palm turns toward body.

**c.** Turn the head to look left and step toward the left with the left foot. Sweep hands forward and out in a circle.

**d.** Bend both knees evenly, push left hand left, and extend right arm back, with the body's weight on both legs.

**End Position**   Right foot points forward and the left foot points left. The head turns left. The left hand pushes to the side, and the right fingers form a beak. Knees are bent evenly.

*Intention:* Push with the left arm, grasp with the right arm, and feel the body's weight even on both legs.

*Attention:* Relax, breathe, feel the earth, and do nothing extra. Attend to how you feel inside.

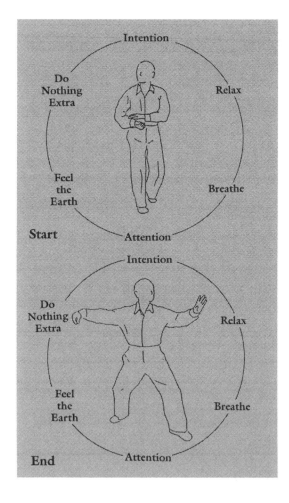

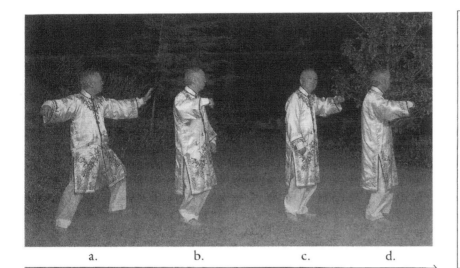

a.   b.   c.   d.

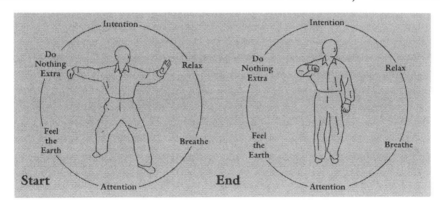

**Start**   **End**

## Movement

**a.** Starting position is the end position from Diagonal Single Whip.

**b.** Shift body weight to the right leg, and move the left foot near the right foot, with left heel up. Both hands make fists. Move the right arm up in front of the body, with the fist at shoulder height, and move the left arm down, with fist at waist height. Arm and leg positions are the same as *d*, with right and left interchanged.

**c.** Step with the left foot to the left corner of the room, and move the right foot near the left foot, with right heel up. Shift the body's weight to the left leg. Raise the left arm up in front of the body with the fist to shoulder height, and lower the right arm to the side with the fist to the waist.

**d.** Step with the right foot to the right corner, and move the left foot near the right foot, with the left heel up. Shift the body's weight to the right leg. Raise the right arm up in front of the body with the fist to shoulder height, and lower left arm to the side with fist to waist height.

**End Position**   Right foot turns out 45° and left heel is up. Right fist is in front of chest and the left fist along the side.

*Intention:* Strike with the left arm, deflect with the right arm, and feel the body's weight on the right leg.

*Attention:* Relax, breathe, feel the earth, and do nothing extra. Attend to how you feel inside.

## 35. Diagonal Single Whip

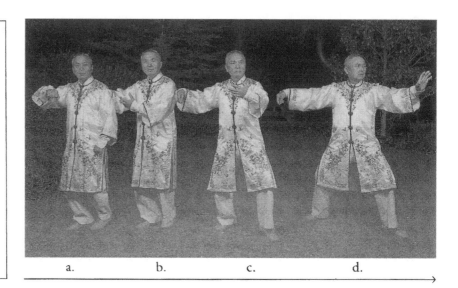

a.　　　b.　　　c.　　　d.

## Movement

**a.** Starting position is the end position from Parting the Wild Horse's Mane.

**b.** Move arms in front of the body. The right fingers form a beak and the left palm turns toward the body.

**c.** Turn the head to look left and step toward the left with the left foot. Sweep hands forward and out in a circle.

**d.** Bend both knees evenly, push left hand left, and extend right arm back, with the body's weight on both legs.

**End Position** Right foot points forward and the left foot points left. The head turns left. The left hand pushes to the side, and the right fingers form a beak. Knees are bent evenly.

*Intention:* Push with the left arm, grasp with the right arm, and feel the body's weight even on both legs.

*Attention:* Relax, breathe, feel the earth, and do nothing extra. Attend to how you feel inside.

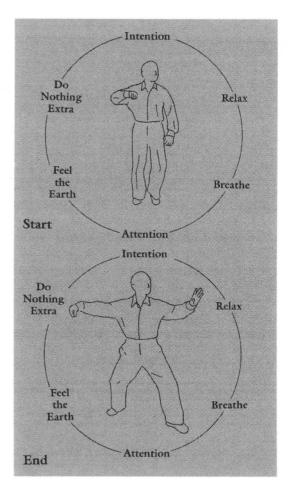

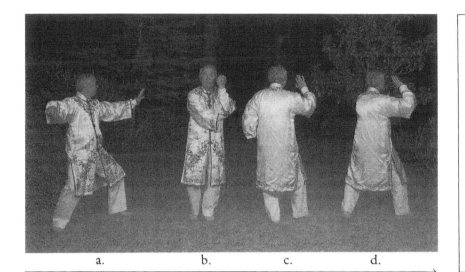

a.   b.   c.   d.

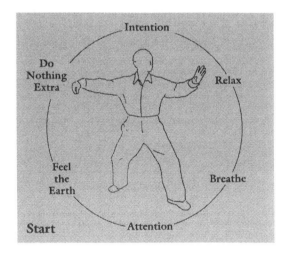

Intention

Do Nothing Extra

Relax

Feel the Earth

Breathe

Start — Attention

## Movement (First Punch)

**a.** Starting position is the end position from Diagonal Single Whip.

**b.** Turn the body and the left foot right 45°. Shift weight to the left leg and move the right foot with heel up near the left foot. Make a fist with the left hand, and place the right hand under the left elbow, with palm out.

**c.** Turn the body right 135° (three-eighths), and step forward with the right foot. Move the right hand toward the temple, and lower the left fist to the waist.

**d.** Bend both knees to shift the body's weight evenly on both legs. Raise the right hand up to temple height and punch with the left arm forward, fist up. This is the same as the end position of the Fourth Punch with right and left interchanged.

*continued*

# Work the Shuttle in the Clouds

🌿

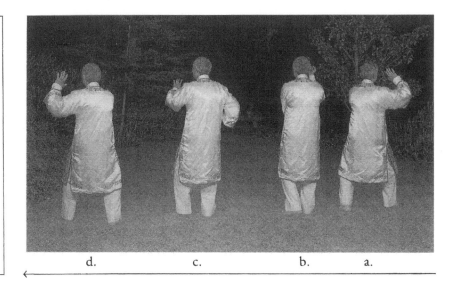

d.          c.          b.          a.

## Movement (Second Punch)

**a.** Start from the end position *d* of the First Punch.

**b.** Turn the body left 90°, shifting the weight to the right leg and moving the left foot near the right foot. Make a fist with the right hand, and place the left hand under the right elbow.

**c.** Step forward with left foot. Move the left hand toward the temple and lower the right fist to the waist.

**d.** Bend both knees to shift the body's weight evenly on both legs. Punch forward with right fist. This is the same as the end position of the Fourth Punch.

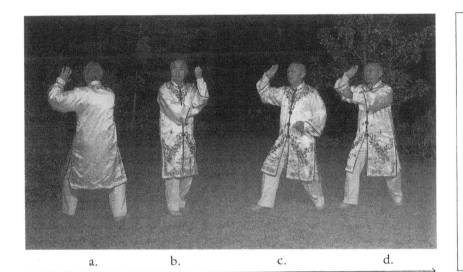

a.　　　　b.　　　　c.　　　　d.

## Work the Shuttle in the Clouds

### Movement (Third Punch)

**a.** Start from the end position *d* of the Second Punch.

**b.** Turn the body and left foot right 90°. Shift weight to the left leg and move the right foot, with heel up, near the left foot. Make a fist with the left hand, and place the right hand under the left elbow, with palm out.

**c.** Turn the body right 180° and step forward with the right foot. Move the right hand toward the temple and lower the left fist to the waist.

**d.** Bend both knees to shift the body's weight evenly on both legs. Punch forward with the left fist. This is the same as the end position of the Fourth Punch with right and left interchanged.

*continued*

## Work the Shuttle in the Clouds

🔥

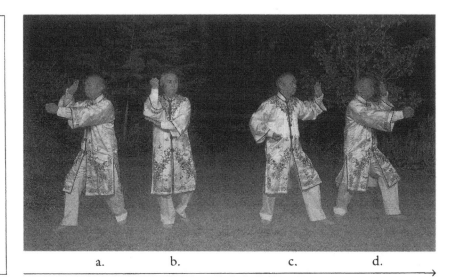

a.  b.  c.  d.

## Movement (Fourth Punch)

**a.** Start from the end position *d* of the Third Punch.

**b.** Turn body left 90°, shift weight to the right leg, and move the left foot, heel up, near the right foot. Make a fist with the right hand, and place the left hand under the right elbow, palm out.

**c.** Step forward with the left foot. Move the left hand toward the temple and the lower right fist to the waist.

**d.** Bend both knees to shift the body's weight evenly on both legs. Punch forward with right fist.

**End Position** Left foot points forward and right foot turns out 60°. The left hand covers the temple with the palm facing out, and the right arm extends forward with a fist.

*Intention:* Punch with right arm, deflect with left arm, and feel body weight even on both legs.

*Attention:* Relax, breathe, feel the earth, and do nothing extra. Attend to how you feel inside.

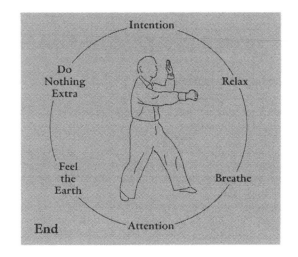

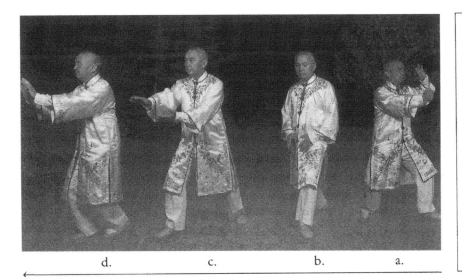

d.       c.       b.       a.

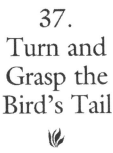

# 37.
# Turn and Grasp the Bird's Tail

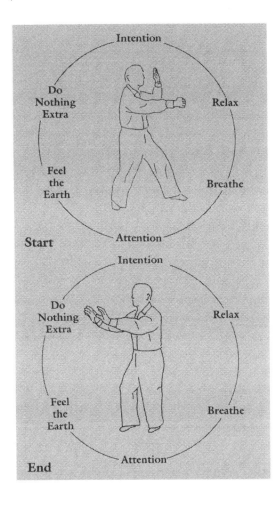

## Movement

**a.** Starting position is the end position from Work the Shuttle in the Clouds.

**b.** Turn the left foot 45° and the body toward the right 90°. Move the right foot near the left foot. Open the right fist and lower both hands. Step forward with the right foot. Bring both hands in front with the right over the left, left palm down and right palm up.

**c.** Bring arms to the left side. Shift weight to the left leg, rest on heel, and lift with toes up.

**d.** Step forward with the right foot and move the left foot behind the right foot, with the left heel up. Push both palms forward with weight evenly distributed on both legs.

**End Position**   Both feet point forward and left foot is behind the right foot. Knees are bent. Hands push forward.

*Intention:* Push with both arms and feel the body's weight on both legs.

*Attention:* Relax, breathe, feel the earth, and do nothing extra. Attend to how you feel inside.

# 38. Single Whip

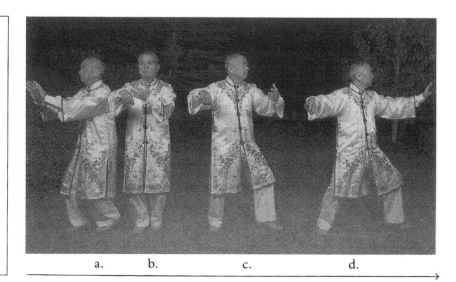

a.　　b.　　c.　　d.

## Movement

**a.** Starting position is the end position from Turn and Grasp the Bird's Tail.

**b.** Turn body and the right foot 45° toward the left. Shift weight to the right leg. Bring both hands in front of the body. Right fingers form a beak and the left palm turns toward the body.

**c.** Turn head toward the left, and turn left foot and step left with the left foot. Move hands out in a circle.

**d.** Bend both knees, lowering the body slightly. Push the left hand toward the left and extend the right arm toward the right.

**End Position**　Right foot points forward and left foot points left. The head turns left and the left hand pushes to the side. The right hand forms a beak; knees are bent evenly.

*Intention:* Push left arm, grasp right arm, and feel body weight even on both legs.

*Attention:* Relax, breathe, feel the earth, and do nothing extra. Attend to how you feel inside.

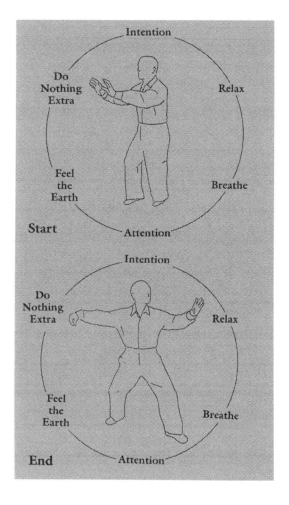

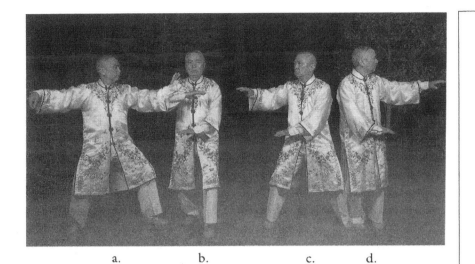

a.　　　b.　　　c.　　　d.

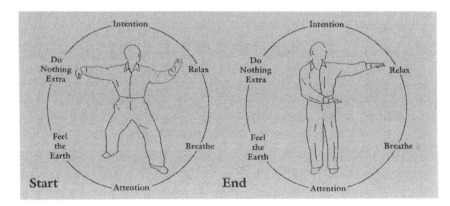

**Start**　Intention · Do Nothing Extra · Relax · Feel the Earth · Breathe · Attention

**End**　Intention · Do Nothing Extra · Relax · Feel the Earth · Breathe · Attention

## Movement

**a.** Starting position is the end position from Single Whip.

**b.** Turn right foot out 45° and shift weight to the right leg. Move the left foot in front, heel up. Bring hands in front of the body with palms down. The right hand is chest-height and the left hand, hip-level.

**c.** Step toward left side with the left foot and turn the right foot parallel to the left foot. Turn the head to look right. Move the right hand toward the right side at shoulder height and the left hand in front of the right hip, palms down. Keep weight even on both legs and bend knees slightly.

**d.** Bring right foot near the left foot. Raise the left hand up and across to shoulder height. Move the right hand down to hip level with body weight even on both legs.

**End Position**　Head turns toward left. Feet are parallel and knees bent evenly. The left arm extends toward the left at shoulder height, palm down, and the right arm is in front of the body near the left hip, palm down.

*Intention:* Sweep with left arm, deflect with right arm, and feel the body's weight on both legs.

*Attention:* Relax, breathe, feel the earth, and do nothing extra. Attend to how you feel inside.

107

## 40. Single Whip Down

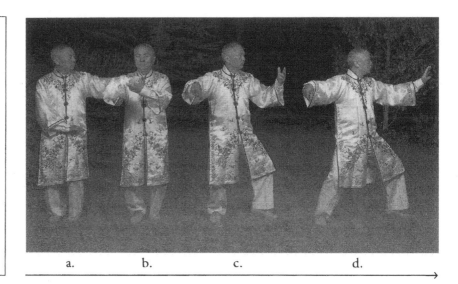

a.  b.  c.  d.

## Movement (First Part)

**a.** Starting position is the end position from Wave Hands Like Clouds.

**b.** Turn the head to look forward, and shift weight to the right leg. Bring both hands in front of the body. The right hand forms a beak and the left palm turns toward the body.

**c.** Turn the head toward the left. Turn the left foot and step left. Move the hands out in a circle.

**d.** Bend both knees, lowering the body slightly. Push toward the left with the left hand, and extend the right arm toward the right with the body's weight even on both legs.

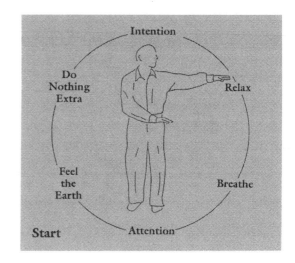

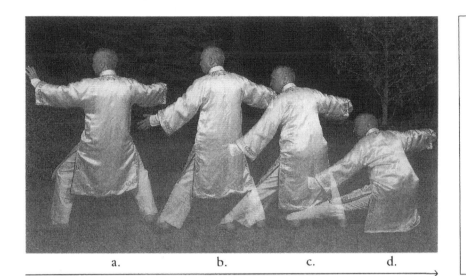

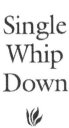

## Single Whip Down

a.      b.      c.      d.

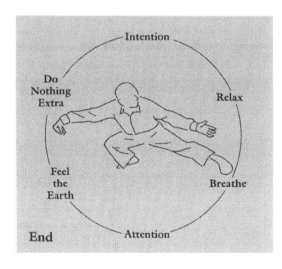

## Movement (Second Part)

**a.** Start from *d* above.

**b.** Shift weight to the left leg, and take a small step to the right with the right foot.

**c.** Turn left foot toward the right 90° with both feet parallel. Turn the body toward the left slightly and lower the body on the right leg with left leg extended.

**d.** Bring the left arm down parallel to the left leg with the palm facing right. Raise the right arm up with hand in a beak.

**End Position**   Feet are parallel, the left leg fully extended and the right knee bent. The head turns toward the left. The left palm faces the front and the right hand forms a beak. Arms extend parallel the legs.

*Intention:* Pull with left arm, grasp with right arm, and feel the body's weight on the right leg.

*Attention:* Relax, breathe, feel the earth, and do nothing extra. Attend to how you feel inside.

## 41.
## Golden Rooster Stands on One Leg

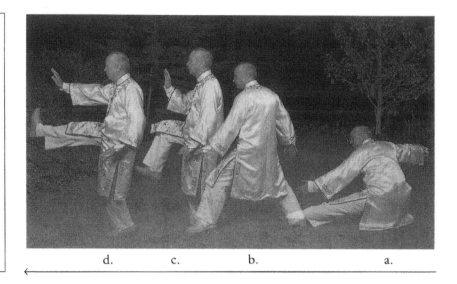

d.       c.       b.       a.

## Movement (First Part)

**a.** Starting position is the end position from Single Whip Down.

**b.** Turn the left foot out 120° and raise the body up.

**c.** Shift weight to the left leg. Bring the right knee up and the right hand in front, chest-height with palm facing forward. Lower the left hand to your side, waist-height with palm facing down.

**d.** Stand on left leg with the knee slightly bent. Push the right heel and right palm forward to complete the first of three arm–leg pushes. The position is the same as *d* in the third part of this movement.

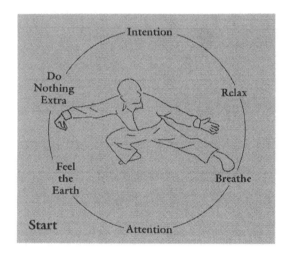

110

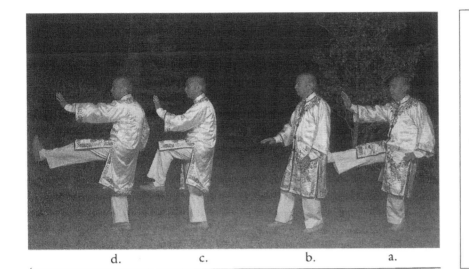

d.       c.       b.       a.

## Golden Rooster Stands on One Leg

## Movement (Second Part)

**a.** Start from the *d* position above.

**b.** Step down with the right foot, turning 30° out. Turn the right palm up and bring it toward the waist.

**c.** Shift weight to the right leg. Bring the left knee up and the left hand in front of the body, chest-height with palm facing forward.

**d.** Stand on the right leg with the knee slightly bent. Push left heel and left palm forward to complete the second of three arm–leg pushes. The position is the same as *d* in the first part with right and left interchanged.

*continued*

# Golden Rooster Stands on One Leg

🔥

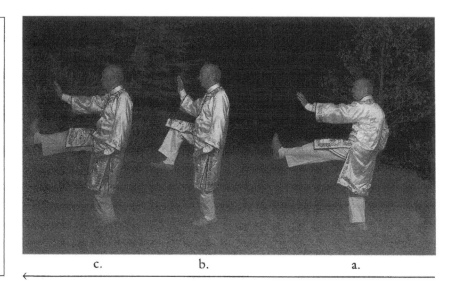

c.  b.  a.

## Movement (Third Part)

**a.** Start from *d* above.

**b.** Step down with the left foot turning 30° out. Turn the left palm up and bring it toward the waist. Shift your weight to the left leg and bring the right knee up and the right hand in front, chest-height with palm facing forward.

**c.** Stand on the left leg with the knee slightly bent. Push the right heel and right palm forward to complete the movement.

**End Position** Left foot turns 30° out with the knee bent. The right leg extends forward, the right palm is in front of the right shoulder, and the left palm is near the waist on the left.

*Intention:* Push with the right arm, pull with the left arm, push with the right leg, and feel the body's weight on the left leg.

*Attention:* Relax, breathe, feel the earth, and do nothing extra. Attend to how you feel inside.

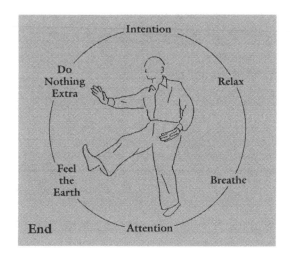

112

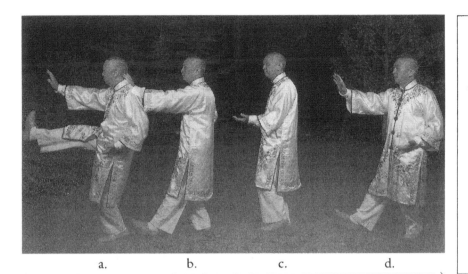

a.　　　b.　　　c.　　　d.

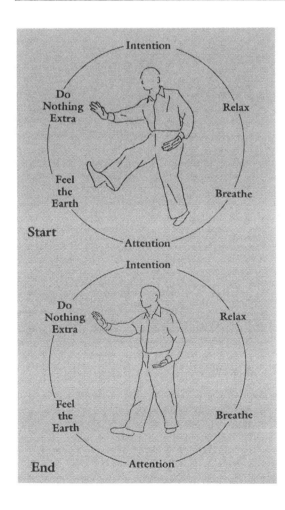

Start

End

## Movement

**a.** Starting position is the end position from Golden Rooster Stands on One Leg.

**b.** Step back with your right foot out 45°. Shift your weight to the right leg and lift up your left toes. Turn the right palm up and pull it back to the waist. Bring the left hand up and push it forward.

**c.** Bring the left foot near the body. Begin to bring the right hand up. Turn the left palm up and bring it down to the waist.

**d.** Step back with your left foot out 45°. Shift weight to the left leg and lift your right toes up. Push the right hand forward and pull the left hand to the waist, palm up.

**End Position**　Left foot turns out 45° and right foot rests on heel. Right hand extends forward with palm out and left hand is along waist with palm up.

*Intention:* Push with right arm, pull with left arm, and feel the body's weight on the left leg.

*Attention:* Relax, breathe, feel the earth, and do nothing extra. Attend to how you feel inside.

113

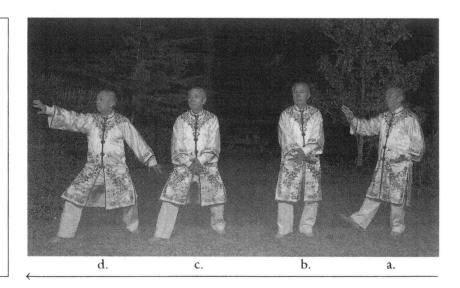

# 43.
## Slanted Palms Flying

d.  c.  b.  a.

## Movement

**a.** Starting position is the end position from Step Back to Repulse the Monkey.

**b.** Turn the left foot and the body 45°. Bring the right foot near the left foot with toes pointing out 45°. Bring both hands in front of the body, with the left wrist above the right wrist. Shift weight to the left leg.

**c.** Step 45° toward the right. Shift weight to both legs with bent knees.

**d.** Sweep arms outward, raising the right arm to shoulder height and the left arm to hip level with palms facing back.

**End Position**  Both feet turn out 45° and knees are bent. Extend both arms along sides, slanted, with palms facing back.

*Intention:* Sweep with right arm, deflect with left arm, and feel the body's weight on both legs.

*Attention:* Relax, breathe, feel the earth, and do nothing extra. Attend to how you feel inside.

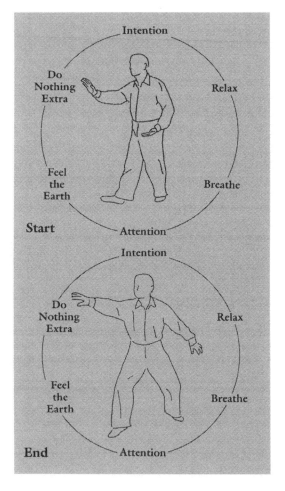

114

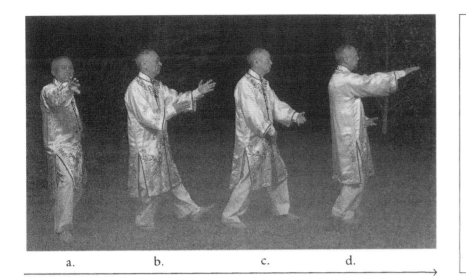

a.  b.  c.  d.

## 44. Raise Right and Left Hands

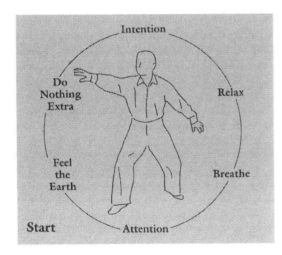

Intention

Do Nothing Extra

Relax

Feel the Earth

Breathe

Start   Attention

## Movement (First Part)

**a.** Starting position is the end position from Slanted Palms Flying.

**b.** Shift weight to the right leg. Bring the left foot in front of the hip. Rest on heel. Move both arms forward, palms in.

**c.** Step down with left foot forward. Lower the left hand with palm up and lower the right hand with palm down.

**d.** Shift the body's weight to the left leg. Bring the right foot near the left foot along the side with the heel up. Raise the right arm and lower the left hand in front of the body. Arm and leg positions are the same as shown in *d* in the second part of this movement, with right and left interchanged.

*continued*

115

# Raise Right and Left Hands

❧

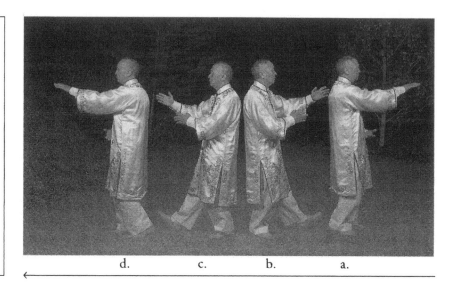

d.　　　c.　　　b.　　　a.

## Movement (Second Part)

**a.** Start from the end position of the first part of this movement.

**b.** Step back with right foot. Lift up the left toes and shift weight to the right leg. Lower the right hand and move the left arm forward along the sides in front of the body, palms in.

**c.** Turn body toward the right 180° and turn on the heel of your left foot 135°. Step down with the left foot. Shift weight to the left leg, and move the right foot slightly to the side, in front of the hip and rest on the heel. Lower the left hand and move the right arm forward.

**d.** Step down on the right foot and shift the body's weight to the right leg. Bring the left foot near the right foot along the side with the heel up. Raise the left arm and lower the right hand in front of the body.

**End Position**　Left foot is behind the right foot along the side, with the left heel up. The left hand points forward at shoulder height, with palm down, and the right hand is in front of the body, palm up.

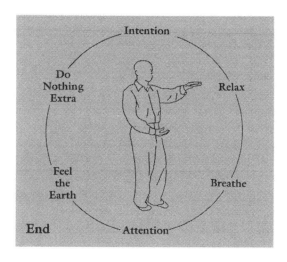

*Intention:* Push with left arm, block with right arm, and feel the body's weight on the right leg.

*Attention:* Relax, breathe, feel the earth, and do nothing extra. Attend to how you feel inside.

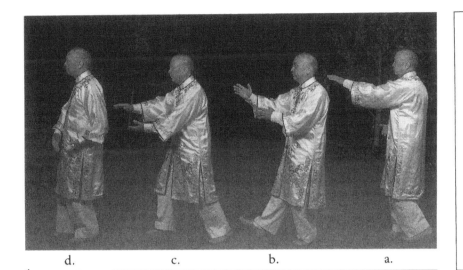

d.    c.    b.    a.

## 45. Step Up with Flying Arm

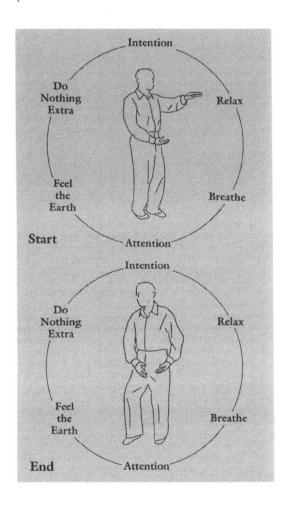

Intention
Do Nothing Extra
Relax
Feel the Earth
Breathe
Start
Attention

Intention
Do Nothing Extra
Relax
Feel the Earth
Breathe
End
Attention

## Movement

**a.** Starting position is the end position from Raise Right and Left Hands.

**b.** Step back with the left foot, toes turned out 45°. Shift the body's weight to the left leg and lift up the right toes. Lower the left hand and move the right arm forward along the sides in front of the body with palms in.

**c.** Step forward with right foot, and reach forward with both hands, right above left, right palm down and left palm up.

**d.** Shift weight to the left leg. Bring the right foot back near the left foot with the right heel up. Pull both hands near the body, waist level along the left side with palms facing each other.

**End Position**   The left foot is 45° out and the right heel up. The right arm crosses the body at 45° and palms face each other.

*Intention:* Deflect down with the right arm, pull with left arm, and feel the body's weight on the left leg.

*Attention:* Relax, breathe, feel the earth, and do nothing extra. Attend to how you feel inside.

117

# 46.
# Fan across Shoulder

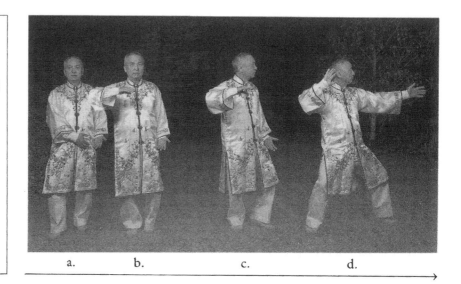

a.    b.         c.         d.

## Movement

**a.** Starting position is the end position from Step Up with Flying Arm.

**b.** Step forward with the right foot and bring left foot near the right foot. Lift up the left heel and shift weight to the right leg. Raise the right elbow to shoulder height, palm down.

**c.** Turn the head to look left. Turn the left foot and left hand toward the left.

**d.** Step with left foot toward the left. Raise the left hand to shoulder height with fingers pointing left, and bring your right hand up to temple level with palm out.

**End Position**   Left foot turns 90° out and right foot points forward. Left hand points left at shoulder level, and right hand covers the head at temple height.

*Intention:* Push out with the left arm, pull back with the right arm, and feel the body's weight on both legs.

*Attention:* Relax, breathe, feel the earth, and do nothing extra. Attend to how you feel inside.

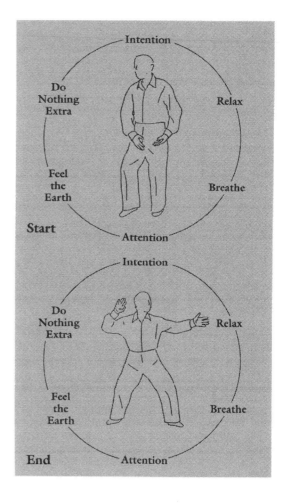

**118**

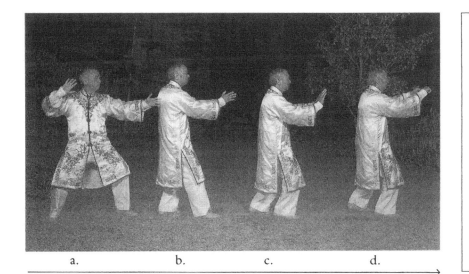

a.  b.  c.  d.

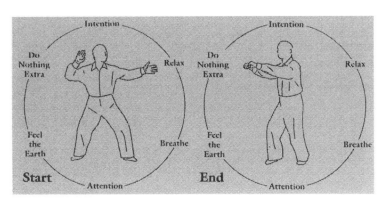

Start    End

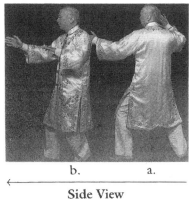

b.  a.

**Side View**

## Movement

**a.** Starting position is the end position from Fan across Shoulder.

**b.** Turn body 90° toward left and left foot out 45°. Shift weight to the left leg and step forward with the right foot, heel up. Move hands to the left side with the right hand in front of the left hand, palms facing left, and fingers pointing forward (see front view).

**c.** Step forward with the right foot, and bring the left foot behind right foot with left heel up. Move hands in front of the body and push forward.

**d.** Shift weight to left leg. Step forward with the right foot and bring the left foot behind right foot with left heel up. Make fists and move them to the sides and forward in a circle. The fists face each other with knuckles up and not touching.

**End Position**  Fists are in front of the body, shoulder-height, not touching. Thumbs face each other and elbows and knees are bent. The right foot is in front of the left foot.

*Intention:* Strike with both arms and feel the body's weight on both legs.

*Attention:* Relax, breathe, feel the earth, and do nothing extra. Attend to how you feel inside.

119

## 48. Firing Cannon into the Sky

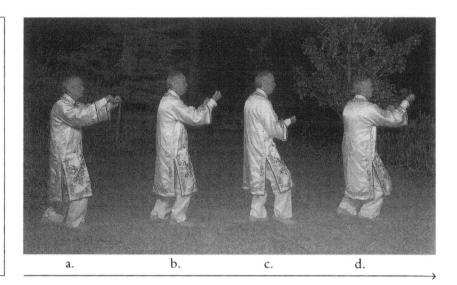

a.  b.  c.  d.

## Movement

**a.** Starting position is the end position from Push and Box Ears.

**b.** Shift weight to the left leg. Turn fists so that fingers face you.

**c.** Lower fists near the body, and lower the left fist slightly, ready to punch.

**d.** Step forward with the right foot and bring the left foot behind right foot with left heel up. Punch fists slightly upward with the body's weight on both legs.

**End Position** Fists turn up with thumbs out. The right arm is higher and in front of the left arm; elbows and knees are bent. The right foot is in front of the left foot.

*Intention:* Punch up with both arms and feel the body's weight on the legs.

*Attention:* Relax, breathe, feel the earth, and do nothing extra. Attend to how you feel inside.

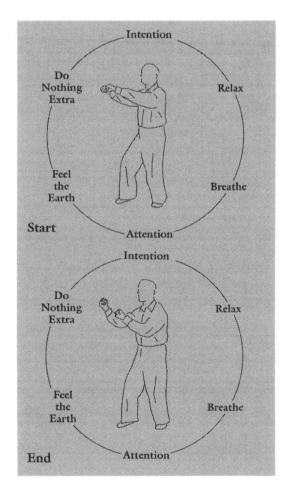

120

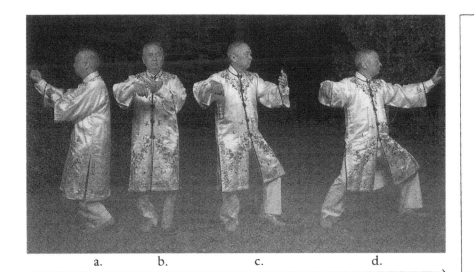

a.    b.    c.    d.

## 49.
## Single
## Whip

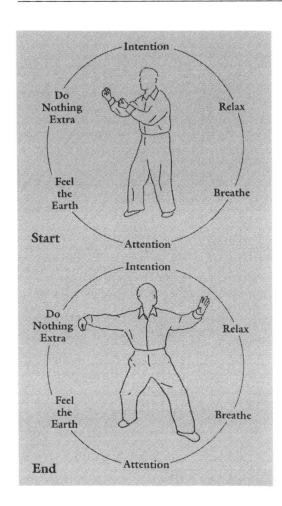

Start

End

## Movement

**a.** Starting position is the end position from Firing Cannon into the Sky.

**b.** Turn body and left foot 90° toward the left. Shift weight to the right leg. Bring both hands in front of the body. The right fingers form a beak and the left palm turns toward the body.

**c.** Turn head toward the left, and turn left foot and step left with the left foot. Move hands out in a circle.

**d.** Bend both knees, lowering the body slightly. Push the left hand toward the left and extend the right arm toward the right.

**End Position**    Right foot points forward and left foot points left. The head turns left and the left hand pushes to the side. The right hand forms a beak; knees are bent evenly.

*Intention:* Push left arm, grasp right arm, and feel body weight even on both legs.

*Attention:* Relax, breathe, feel the earth, and do nothing extra. Attend to how you feel inside.

121

## 50. Wave Hands Like Clouds

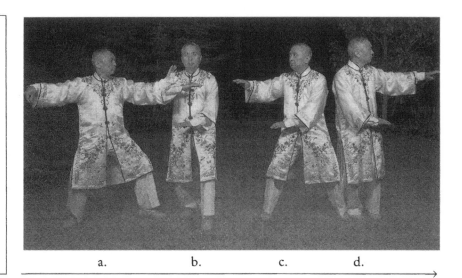

a.  b.  c.  d.

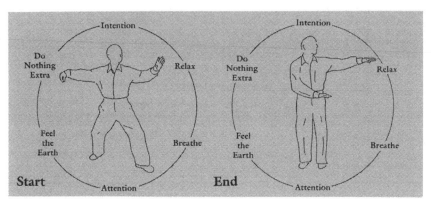

## Movement

**a.** Starting position is the end position from Single Whip.

**b.** Turn right foot out 45° and shift weight to the right leg. Move the left foot in front, with heel up. Bring hands in front of the body with palms down. The right hand is at chest height and left hand hip-level.

**c.** Step toward left side with the left foot and turn the right foot parallel to the left foot. Turn the head to look right. Move the right hand toward the right side at shoulder height and the left hand in front of the right hip, palms down. Keep weight even on both legs and bend knees slightly.

**d.** Bring right foot near the left foot. Raise the left hand up and across to shoulder height. Move the right hand down to hip level with body weight even on both legs.

**End Position**   Head turns toward left. Feet are parallel and knees bent evenly. The left arm extends toward the left at shoulder height, palm down, and the right arm is in front of the body near the left hip, palm down.

*Intention:* Sweep with left arm, deflect with right arm, and feel the body's weight on both legs.

*Attention:* Relax, breathe, feel the earth, and do nothing extra. Attend to how you feel inside.

122

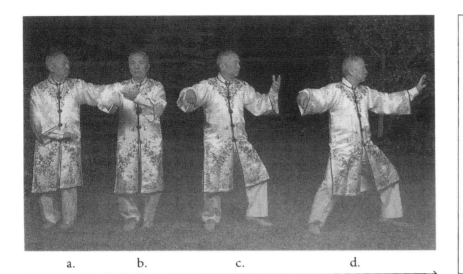

# 51. Single Whip

a.       b.       c.       d.

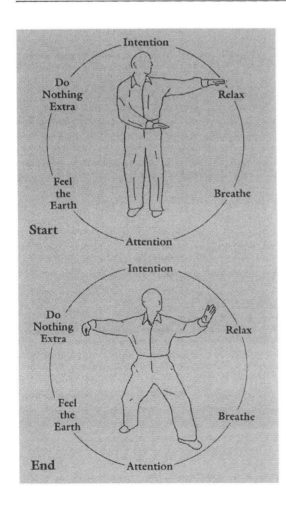

## Movement

**a.** Starting position is the end position from Wave Hands Like Clouds.

**b.** Turn the head to look forward and shift weight to the right leg. Bring both hands in front of the body. Form a beak with the right hand, and turn the left palm toward the body.

**c.** Turn head toward the left, and turn left foot and step left with the left foot. Move hands out in a circle.

**d.** Bend both knees, lowering the body slightly. Push the left hand toward the left and extend the right arm toward the right.

**End Position**   Right foot points forward and left foot points left. The head turns left and the left hand pushes to the side. The right hand forms a beak; knees are bent evenly.

*Intention:* Push left arm, grasp right arm, and feel body weight even on both legs.

*Attention:* Relax, breathe, feel the earth, and do nothing extra. Attend to how you feel inside.

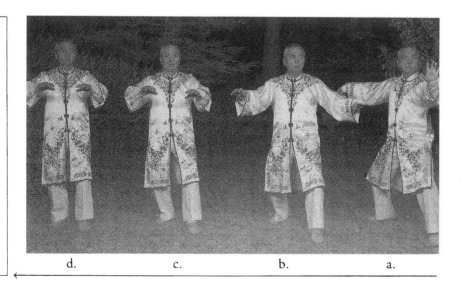

| d. | c. | b. | a. |

## 52. High Pat on Horse

## Movement

**a.** Starting position is the end position from Single Whip.

**b.** Turn the body and the right foot 45° toward the left.

**c.** Shift weight to the right leg and bring the left foot in front of the hip, with heel up. Move both hands in front of the chest, palms down.

**d.** Bend knees and complete the movement with the body's weight on the right leg.

**End Position**  Right foot is out 45° and the left heel up; knees are bent. Hands are in front of the chest, arms in a circle and palms down.

*Intention:* Block with the left arm, hold with the right arm, and feel the body's weight on the right leg.

*Attention:* Relax, breathe, feel the earth, and do nothing extra. Attend to how you feel inside.

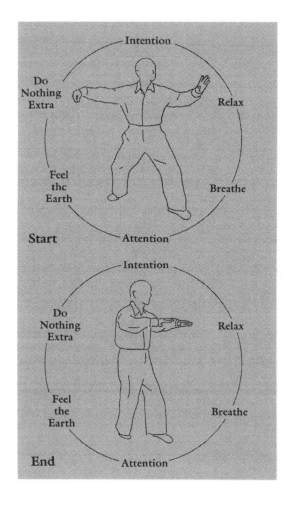

124

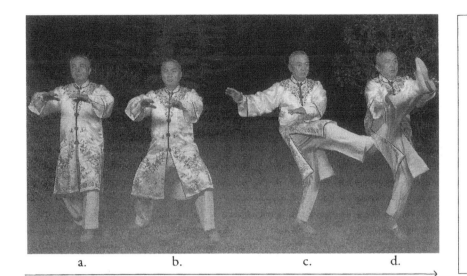

a.    b.    c.    d.

## 53. Wave Cross at Water Lily

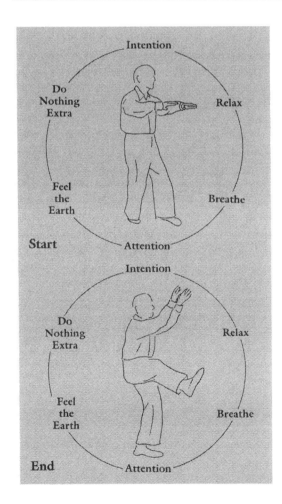

Intention

Do Nothing Extra          Relax

Feel the Earth          Breathe

**Start**     Attention

Intention

Do Nothing Extra          Relax

Feel the Earth          Breathe

**End**     Attention

## Movement

**a.** Starting position is the end position from High Pat on Horse.

**b.** Step toward the left 45° with the left foot, with toes pointing out also 45°. Shift weight evenly on both legs with knees bent.

**c.** Shift weight to left leg and raise right foot up and across the body toward the left side of the body. Move your arms toward the right side.

**d.** Sweep the right foot across in front of the body from left to right, and sweep the palms from right to left brushing your right knee.

**End Position**   Right foot sweeps across clockwise from left to right. Hands circle from right to left, with the left knee bent. The left foot turns 45° out.

*Intention:* Sweep with both arms, kick with the right leg, and feel the body's weight on the left leg.

*Attention:* Relax, breathe, feel the earth, and do nothing extra. Attend to how you feel inside.

125

# 54.
# Fist Pounding Down

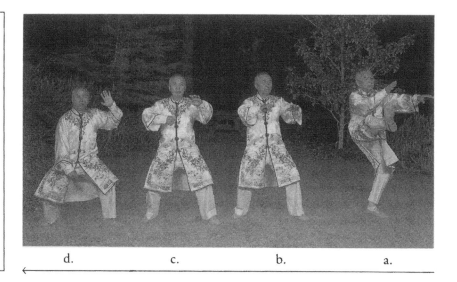

d.    c.    b.    a.

## Movement

**a.** Starting position is the end position from Wave Cross at Water Lily.

**b.** Step with the right foot toward the right rear corner of the room. Shift weight evenly to both legs with knees bent. Make a fist with the right hand in front of body.

**c.** Bring the right fist up slightly, and raise the left hand toward your temple.

**d.** Lower the body and bend the knees slightly. Punch downward with the right fist, with knuckles facing forward, and move the left hand to your temple, with palm facing out.

**End Position**   Feet turn 45° out, knees are bent evenly, and the right hand extends downward with the fist, knuckles out, in front of the body. The left hand is near the temple, palm out.

*Intention:* Punch with right arm, block with left arm, and feel your weight even on both legs.

*Attention:* Relax, breathe, feel the earth, and do nothing extra. Attend to how you feel inside.

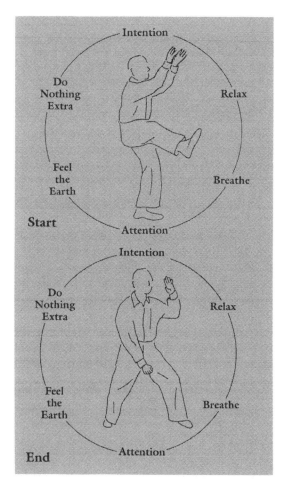

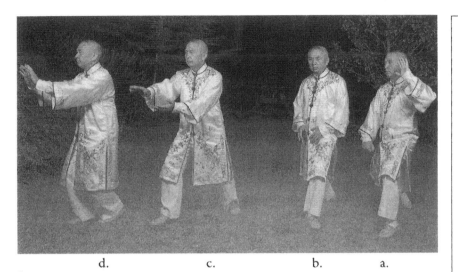

d.    c.    b.    a.

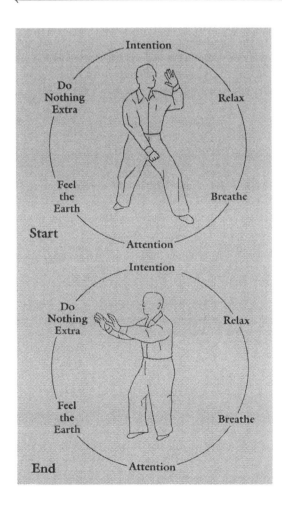

Start

End

## Movement

**a.** Starting position is the end position from Fist Pounding Down.

**b.** Turn the left foot 45° and the body toward the left 90°. Move the right foot near the left foot. Open the right fist and lower both hands. Step forward with the right foot. Bring both hands in front with the right over the left, left palm down and right palm up.

**c.** Bring arms to the left side. Shift weight to the left leg, rest on heel, and lift with toes up.

**d.** Step forward with the right foot and move the left foot behind the right foot, with the left heel up. Push both palms forward with weight evenly distributed on both legs.

**End Position**   Both feet point forward and left foot is behind the right foot. Knees are bent. Hands push forward.

*Intention:* Push with both arms and feel the body's weight on both legs.

*Attention:* Relax, breathe, feel the earth, and do nothing extra. Attend to how you feel inside.

# 56. Single Whip

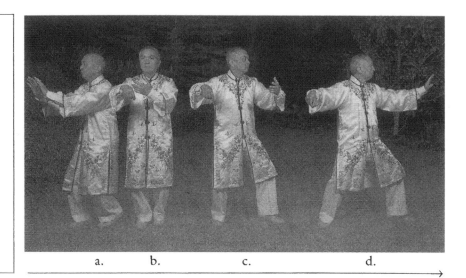

a.　　b.　　　c.　　　　d.

## Movement

**a.** Starting position is the end position from Turn and Grasp the Bird's Tail.

**b.** Turn body and right foot 45° toward the left. Shift weight to the right leg and bring both hands in front of the body. The right hand forms a beak, and the left palm turns toward the body.

**c.** Turn head toward the left, and turn left foot and step left with the left foot. Move hands out in a circle.

**d.** Bend both knees, lowering the body slightly. Push the left hand toward the left and extend the right arm toward the right.

**End Position**　Right foot points forward and left foot points left. The head turns left and the left hand pushes to the side. The right hand forms a beak; knees are bent evenly.

*Intention:* Push left arm, grasp right arm, and feel body weight even on both legs.

*Attention:* Relax, breathe, feel the earth, and do nothing extra. Attend to how you feel inside.

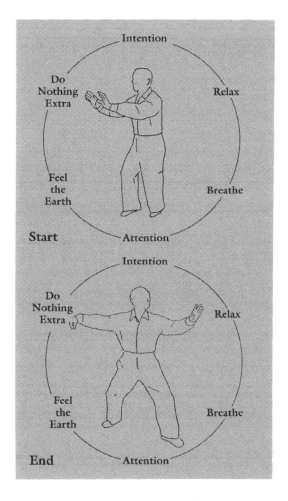

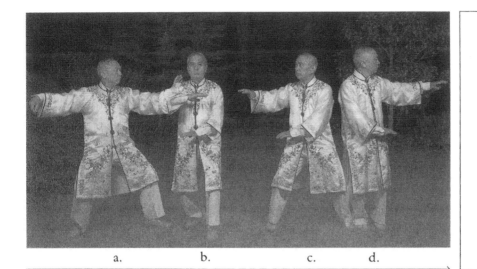

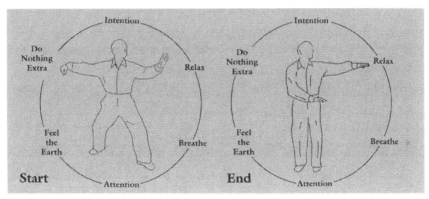

a.    b.    c.    d.

57.
Wave
Hands
Like
Clouds

## Movement

**a.** Starting position is the end position from Single Whip.

**b.** Turn right foot out 45° and shift weight to the right leg. Move the left foot in front, heel up, and bring hands in front of the body with palms down. The right hand is chest-height and left hand hip-level.

**c.** Step toward left side with the left foot and turn the right foot parallel to the left foot. Turn the head to look right. Move the right hand toward the right side at shoulder height and the left hand in front of the right hip, palms down. Keep weight even on both legs and bend knees slightly.

**d.** Bring right foot near the left foot. Raise the left hand up and across to shoulder height. Move the right hand down to hip level with body weight even on both legs.

**End Position** Head turns toward left. Feet are parallel and knees bent evenly. The left arm extends toward the left at shoulder height, palm down, and the right arm is in front of the body near the left hip, palm down.

*Intention:* Sweep with left arm, deflect with right arm, and feel the body's weight on both legs.
*Attention:* Relax, breathe, feel the earth, and do nothing extra. Attend to how you feel inside.

## 58. Single Whip Down

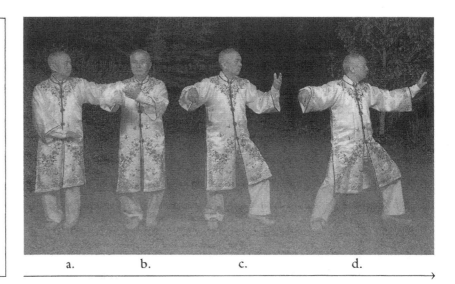

a.  b.  c.  d.

## Movement (First Part)

**a.** Starting position is the end position from Wave Hands Like Clouds.

**b.** Turn the head to look forward, and shift weight to the right leg. Bring both hands in front of the body. The right hand forms a beak and the left palm turns toward the body.

**c.** Turn the head toward the left. Turn the left foot and step left. Move the hands out in a circle.

**d.** Bend both knees, lowering the body slightly. Push toward the left with the left hand, and extend the right arm toward the right with the body's weight even on both legs.

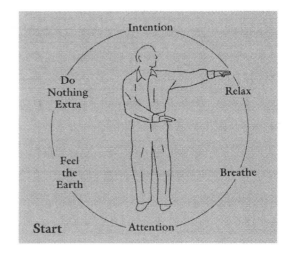

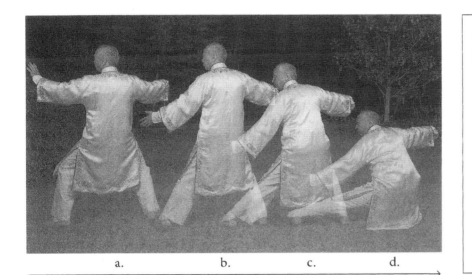

a.  b.  c.  d.

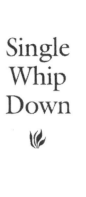

Single
Whip
Down

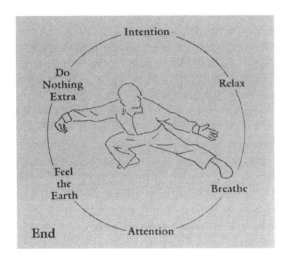

Intention

Do
Nothing
Extra

Relax

Feel
the
Earth

Breathe

End

Attention

## Movement (Second Part)

**a.** Start from *d* above.

**b.** Shift weight to the left leg, and take a small step to the right with the right foot.

**c.** Turn left foot toward the right 90° with both feet parallel. Turn the body toward the left slightly and lower the body on the right leg with left leg extended.

**d.** Bring the left arm down parallel to the left leg with the palm facing right. Raise the right arm up with hand in a beak.

**End Position**   Feet are parallel, the left leg fully extended and the right knee bent. The head turns toward the left. The left palm faces the front and the right hand forms a beak. Arms extend parallel the legs.

*Intention:* Pull with left arm, grasp with right arm, and feel the body's weight on the right leg.

*Attention:* Relax, breathe, feel the earth, and do nothing extra. Attend to how you feel inside.

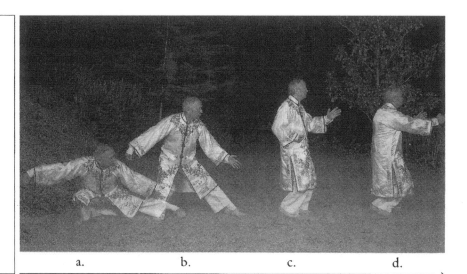

a.　　　　b.　　　　c.　　　　d.

## 59. Step to Reach Seven Stars

## Movement

**a.** Starting position is the end position from Single Whip Down.

**b.** Turn the body toward the left and the left foot out 45°; raise the body up.

**c.** Shift weight to the left leg. With the right foot step behind and along the side of the left foot, with heel up. Make a fist with the right hand and bring it near the body. Bring the left hand in front of the body, palm facing right.

**d.** Bend both knees, lowering the body slightly. Punch forward with the right fist. The left hand is next to the right wrist, with fingers pointing up.

**End Position** Left foot is in front of the right foot, heel up, knees are bent. The right arm extends forward along the side and the left arm bent. The right fist is on the right side and the left palm is near the right forearm, not touching.

*Intention:* Punch with the right arm, block with the left arm, and feel the body's weight on the left leg.

*Attention:* Relax, breathe, feel the earth, and do nothing extra. Attend to how you feel inside.

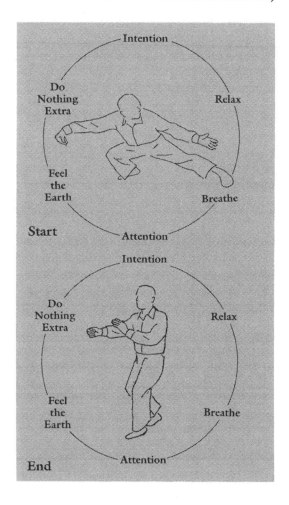

132

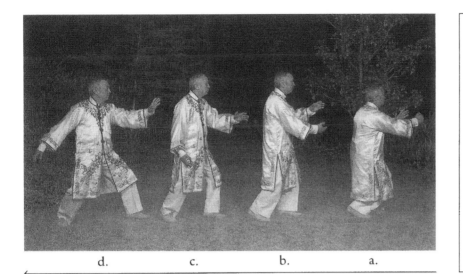

d.　　　c.　　　b.　　　a.

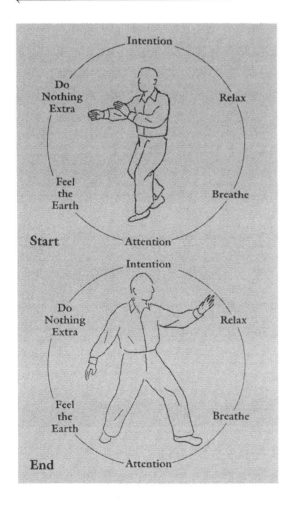

Intention

Do Nothing Extra

Relax

Feel the Earth

Breathe

**Start**

Attention

Intention

Do Nothing Extra

Relax

Feel the Earth

Breathe

**End**

Attention

## Movement

**a.** Starting position is the end position from Step to Reach Seven Stars.

**b.** Step backward with the right foot. Open right fist and raise up the body slightly.

**c.** Put your right foot down with toes pointing 45° out. Move your right arm toward the back and your left arm forward along your side.

**d.** Push the left palm forward and move the right hand backward with your weight on both legs.

**End Position**   Left foot is in front pointing forward and the right foot is out 45°. Knees are bent and the weight is even on both legs. The left palm faces the front and the left arm extends forward and the right palm faces forward and the right arm extends back.

*Intention:* Push forward with the left arm and strike backwards with the right arm. Feel the body's weight on both legs.

*Attention:* Relax, breathe, feel the earth, and do nothing extra. Attend to how you feel inside.

133

## 61. Slant Body to Rock the Moon

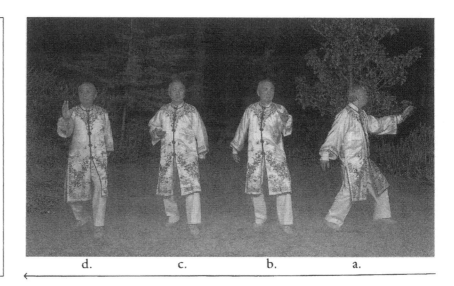

d.    c.    b.    a.

## Movement

**a.** Starting position is the end position from Retreat to Ride the Tiger.

**b.** Turn the body and the right foot toward the right 90°. Shift the body's weight to the right leg and bring the left foot in front of left hip, heel up. Bend your knees.

**c.** Move the right hand forward and lower the left hand. Make a beak with the left hand.

**d.** Push your right palm forward and up, and grasp with your left hand backwards and down along the side.

**End Position**   Right foot is 45° out and the left heel is up in front of the left hip. The right palm pushes forward and the left hand makes a beak, pointing up. The left arm extends backwards.

*Intention:* Push with the right arm and grasp with the left arm. Feel your weight on the right leg.

*Attention:* Relax, breathe, feel the earth, and do nothing extra. Attend to how you feel inside.

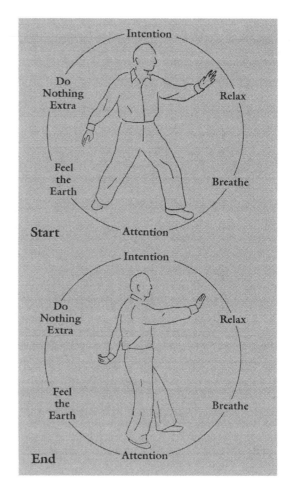

134

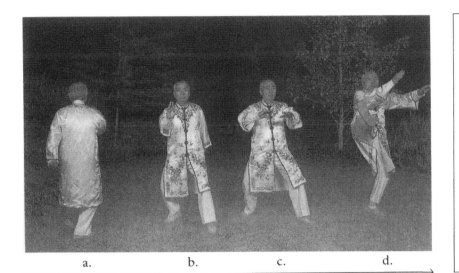

a.        b.        c.        d.

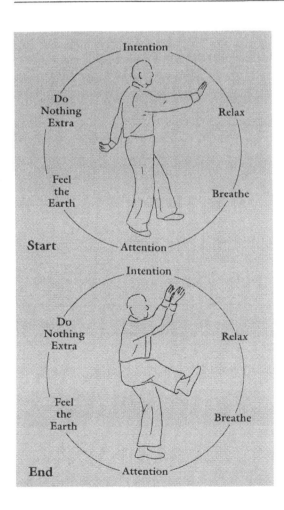

## Movement

**a.** Starting position is the end position from Slant Body to Rock the Moon.

**b.** Lift up the left foot slightly and turn the body 180° toward the right by turning the right foot. Step down with the left foot toward the left 45°. Bend knees and shift the weight evenly on the legs with feet 45° out.

**c.** Move left hand forward, and keep both palms down.

**d.** Shift weight to the left leg, and move the right foot to the left side. Move hands to the right side of the body. Sweep the right foot across in front of the body from left to right and sweep the palms from right to left to brush right knee.

**End Position** The right foot sweeps across from left to right as the hands move from right to left. The left knee is bent and the left foot turns out 45°.

*Intention:* Sweep with both arms, kick with the right leg, and feel the body's weight on the left leg.

*Attention:* Relax, breathe, feel the earth, and do nothing extra. Attend to how you feel inside.

135

## 63. Pulling Bow to Shoot an Arrow

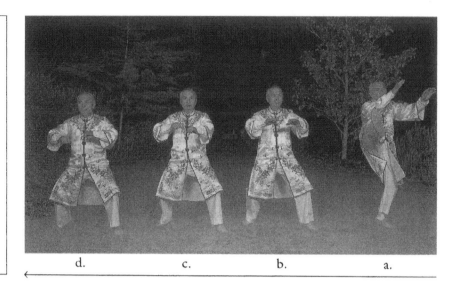

d.        c.        b.        a.

## Movement

**a.** Starting position is the end position from Wave Lotus Foot.

**b.** With right foot step down and back 45° toward the right. Shift the weight evenly to both legs, with knees bent, and bring hands in front of the body.

**c.** Make two fists, knuckles up.

**d.** Circle the right fist toward the body counterclockwise and follow with the left fist circling clockwise. Punch the right fist down slightly at the end of the circle.

**End Position**   Feet turn 45° out, knees are bent evenly, and fists, knuckles up, are in front of the chest. Arms form a circle with the right fist lower and in front of the left fist.

*Intention:* Punch with the right hand, block with left arm, and feel your weight even on both legs.

*Attention:* Relax, breathe, feel the earth, and do nothing extra. Attend to how you feel inside.

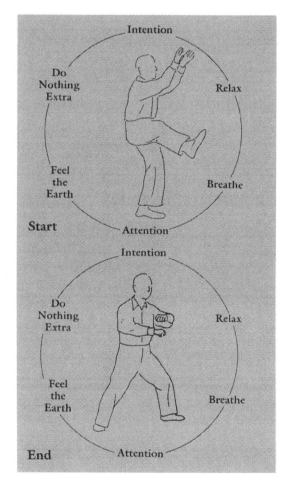

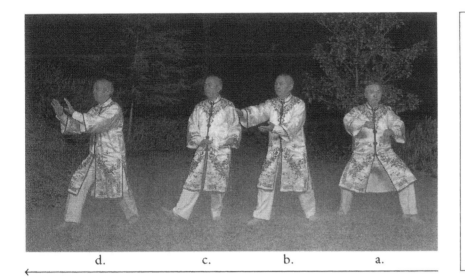

d.    c.    b.    a.

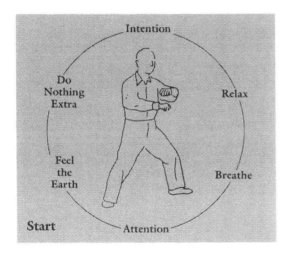

## Movement (First Part)

**a.** Starting position is the end position from Pulling Bow to Shoot an Arrow.

**b.** Shift weight to the left leg and turn the body 45° toward the right. Move the right foot near the body and step right. Move arms forward with the right palm down and left palm up, with weight even on both legs.

**c.** Shift your weight to the left leg and lift up the right toes. Lower your arms to the left side near the body with the right palm down and the left palm up.

**d.** Step down with right foot and push palms forward with the body's weight on both legs.

*continued*

137

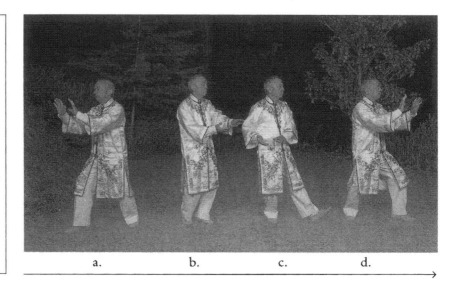

## Right and Left Grasp the Bird's Tail

a.      b.      c.      d.

## Movement (Second Part)

**a.** Start from *d* above.

**b.** Shift weight to the right leg. Turn the left foot 45° left and turn the body left 90°. Shift weight to the left leg and bring the right foot near the left foot. Move hands down in front of the body.

**c.** Step back with the right foot. Shift your weight to the right leg and lift up left toes. Lower your arms to the right side near the body with the left palm down and the right palm up.

**d.** Step down with the left foot and push forward with the body's weight even on both legs.

**End Position**    Left foot points forward and the right foot turns out 60°, with knees bent evenly.

*Intention:* Push with both arms and feel the body's weight even on both legs.

*Attention:* Relax, breathe, feel the earth, and do nothing extra. Attend to how you feel inside.

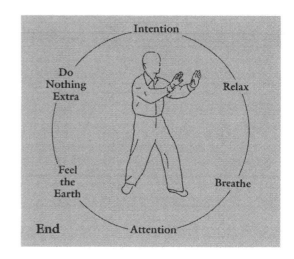

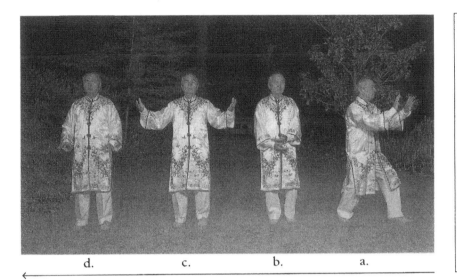

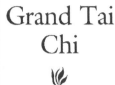

# Grand Tai Chi

d.       c.       b.       a.

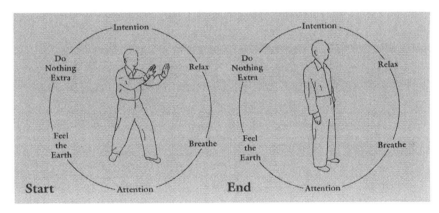

**Starting Position** Left foot points forward and the right foot turns out 60°, with knees bent evenly.

*Intention:* Push with both arms and feel the body's weight evenly on both legs.
*Attention:* Relax, breathe, feel the earth, and do nothing extra. Attend to how you feel inside.

## Movement

a. Starting position is the end position from Right and Left Grasp the Bird's Tail.

b. Turn the body 45° right and move the left foot near the right foot with toes pointing forward and feet parallel. Shift the weight so that it's even on both legs. Lower the arms in front of the body with wrists crossed and palms facing up; knees are slightly bent.

c. Open the arms and raise the hands up and out slowly to temple height.

d. Close the eyes. Turn palms down and lower the arms slowly and evenly to the sides.

**End Position** Feet are parallel, hands along the sides, and knees bent slightly.
*Intention and Attention:* Relax, breathe, feel the earth, and do nothing extra.

Adding the four one-with-nature elements, Grand Tai Chi becomes One-with-Nature Tone Ch'i (see p. 27).

收心養性
身鬆氣通
平意靜心
氣壯身強

祚榮先生囑書

戊辰秋石因

# Index

For more information on tai chi visit the website:
www.taichiculturalcenter.com

Printed in Great Britain
by Amazon